A Day on The Beach

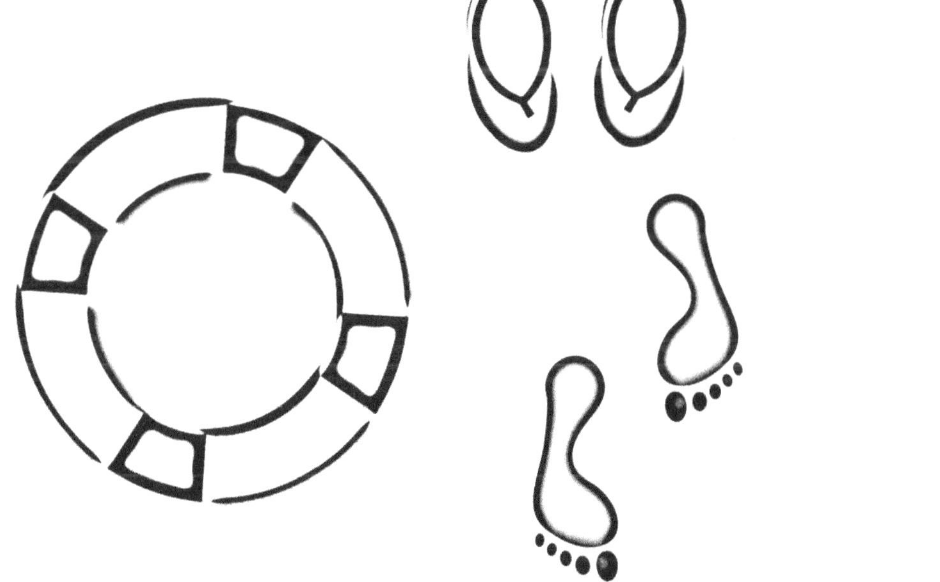

This book belongs to

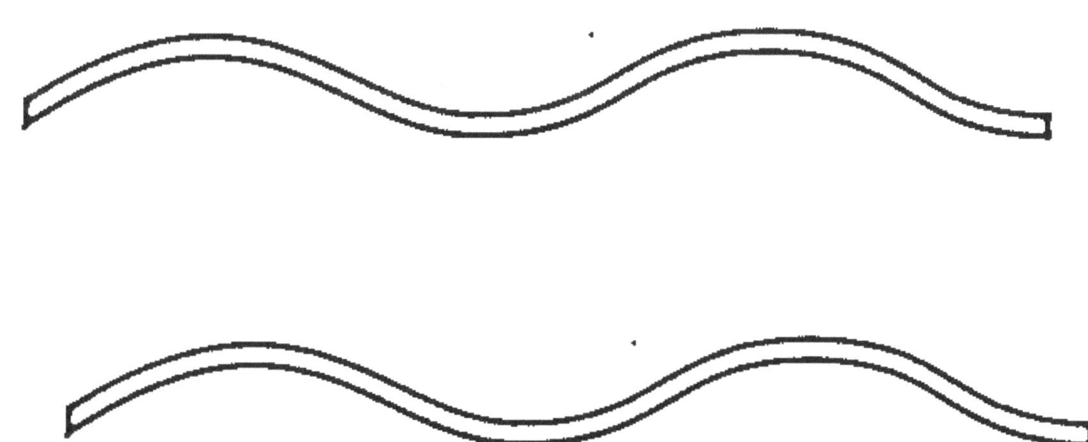

Coloring is a powerful method of relaxation through practicing mindful meditation.

This book contains more than 50 carefully selected , highly detailed coloring pictures featuring various cheerful beach scenes and activities for the sole purpose of helping you practice mindful meditation.

Here are few tips to help you relax:

• Take slow, deep breaths, or try other breathing exercises for relaxation.

• Soak in a warm bath.

• Listen to soothing music.

• Turn off TV and any other unnecessary background noise.

• Enjoy daylight whenever you can.

• Practice mindful meditation, grab your crayons and a sharpener. Sit back and have fun.

Produced by Enchanted Beauty , 2020.

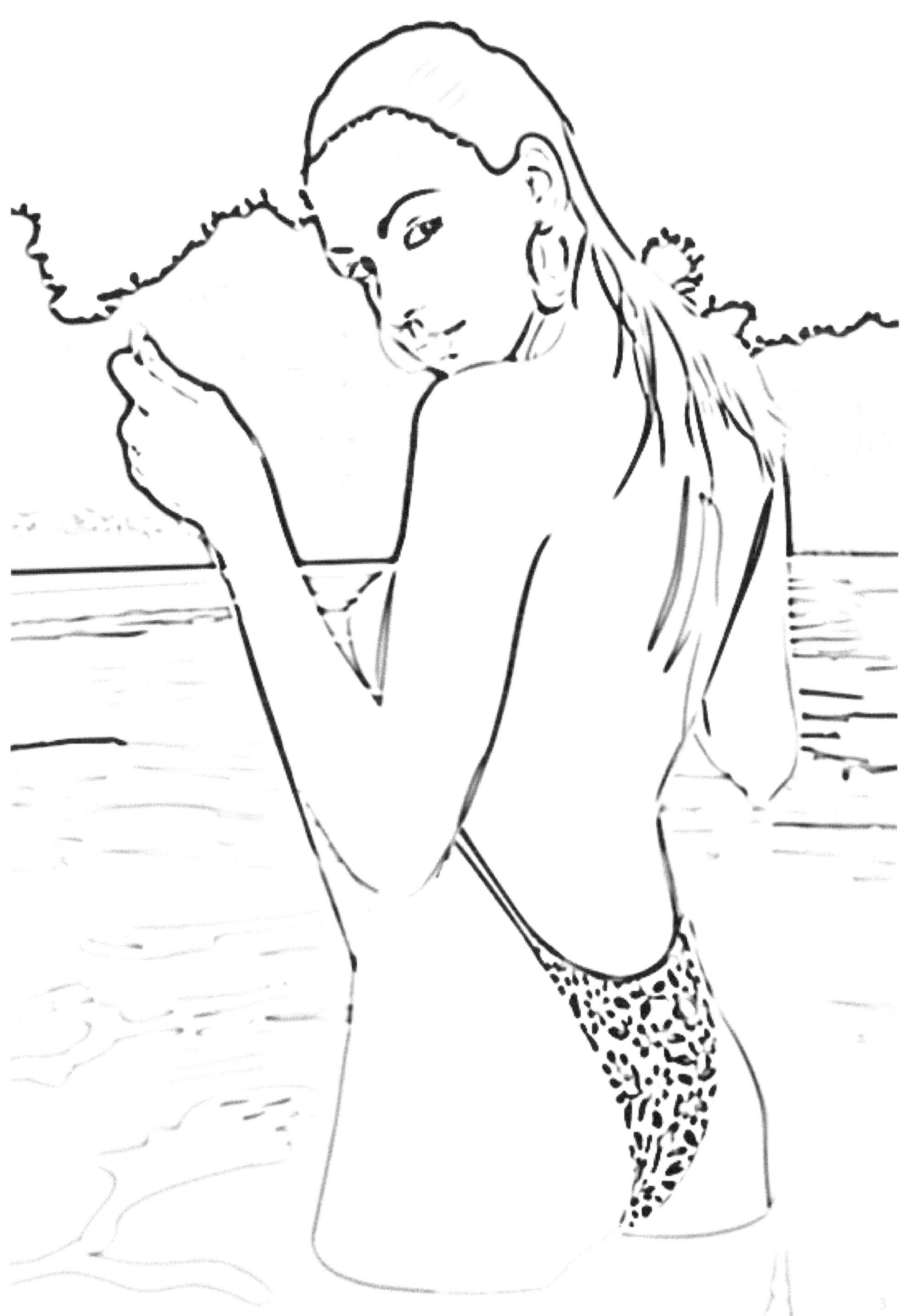

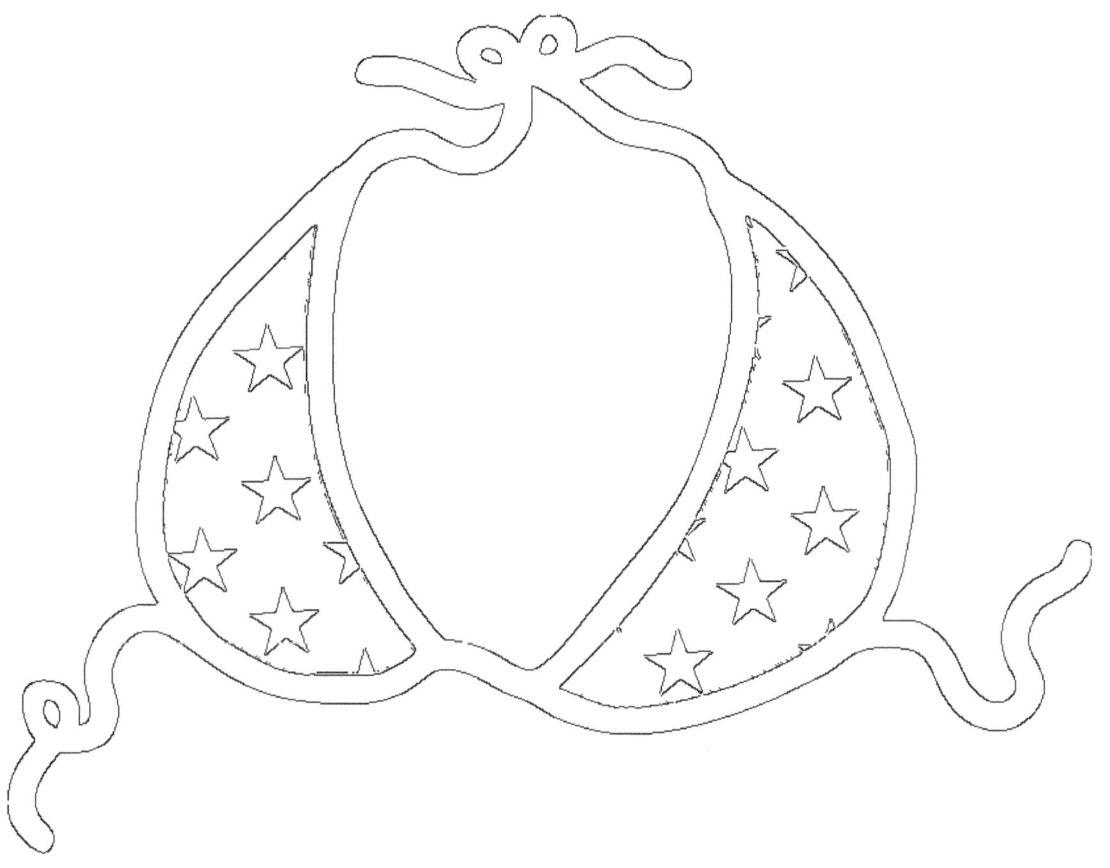

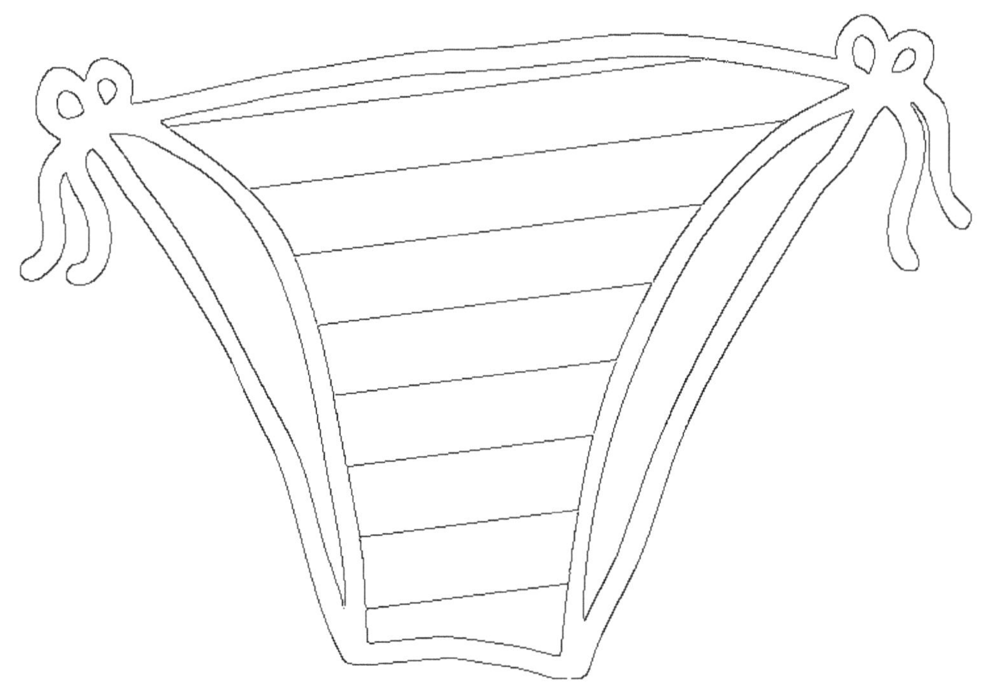

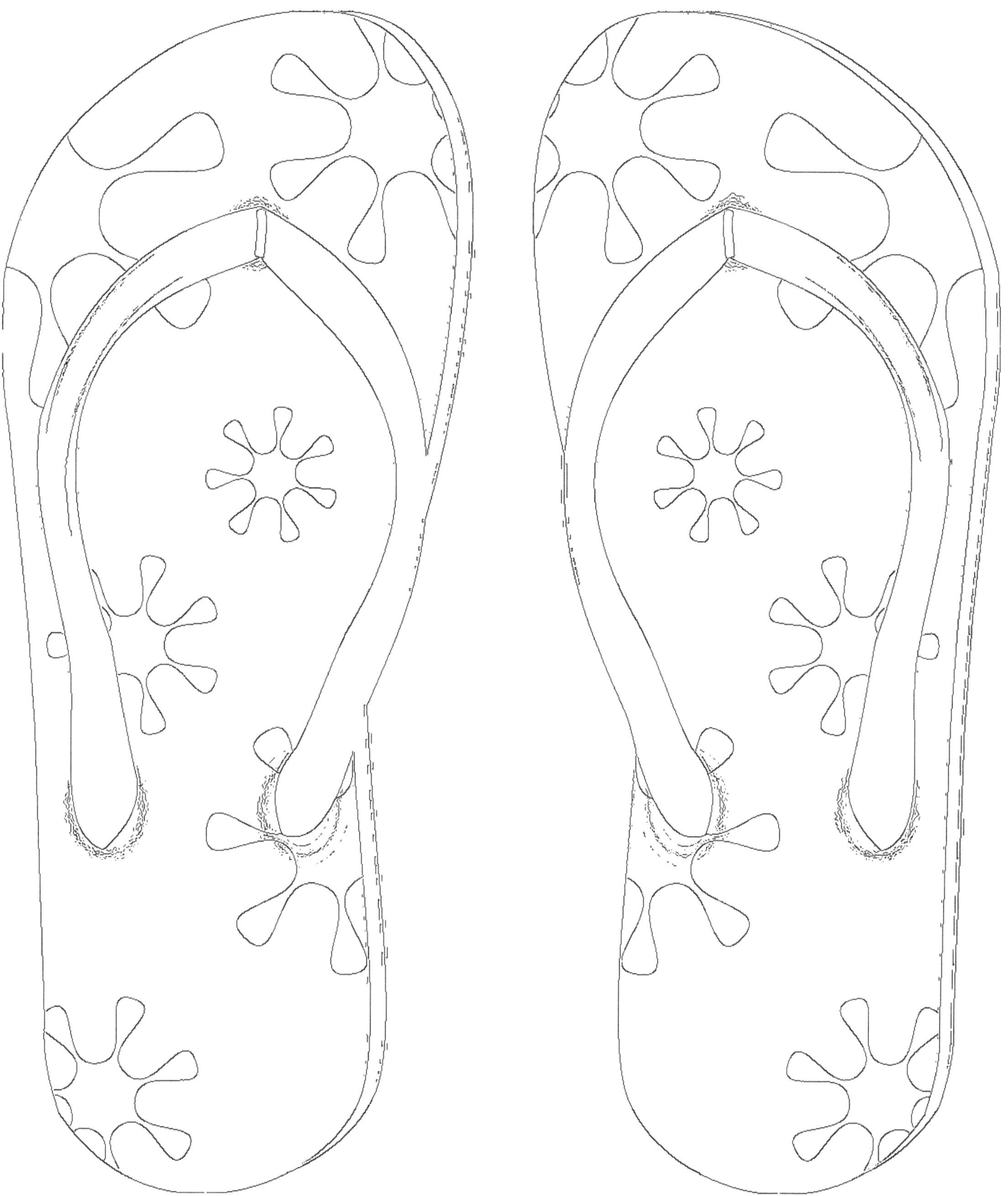

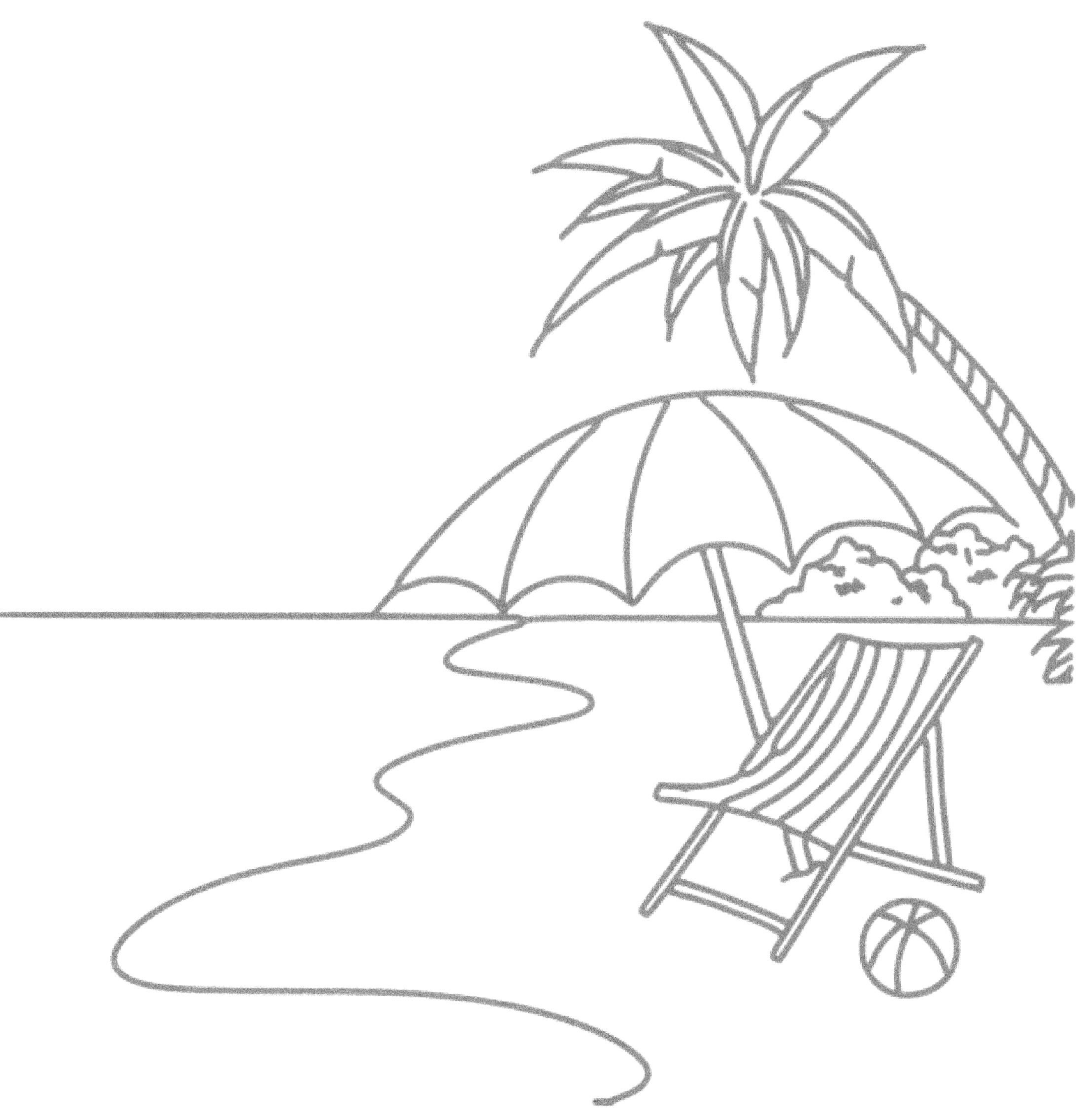

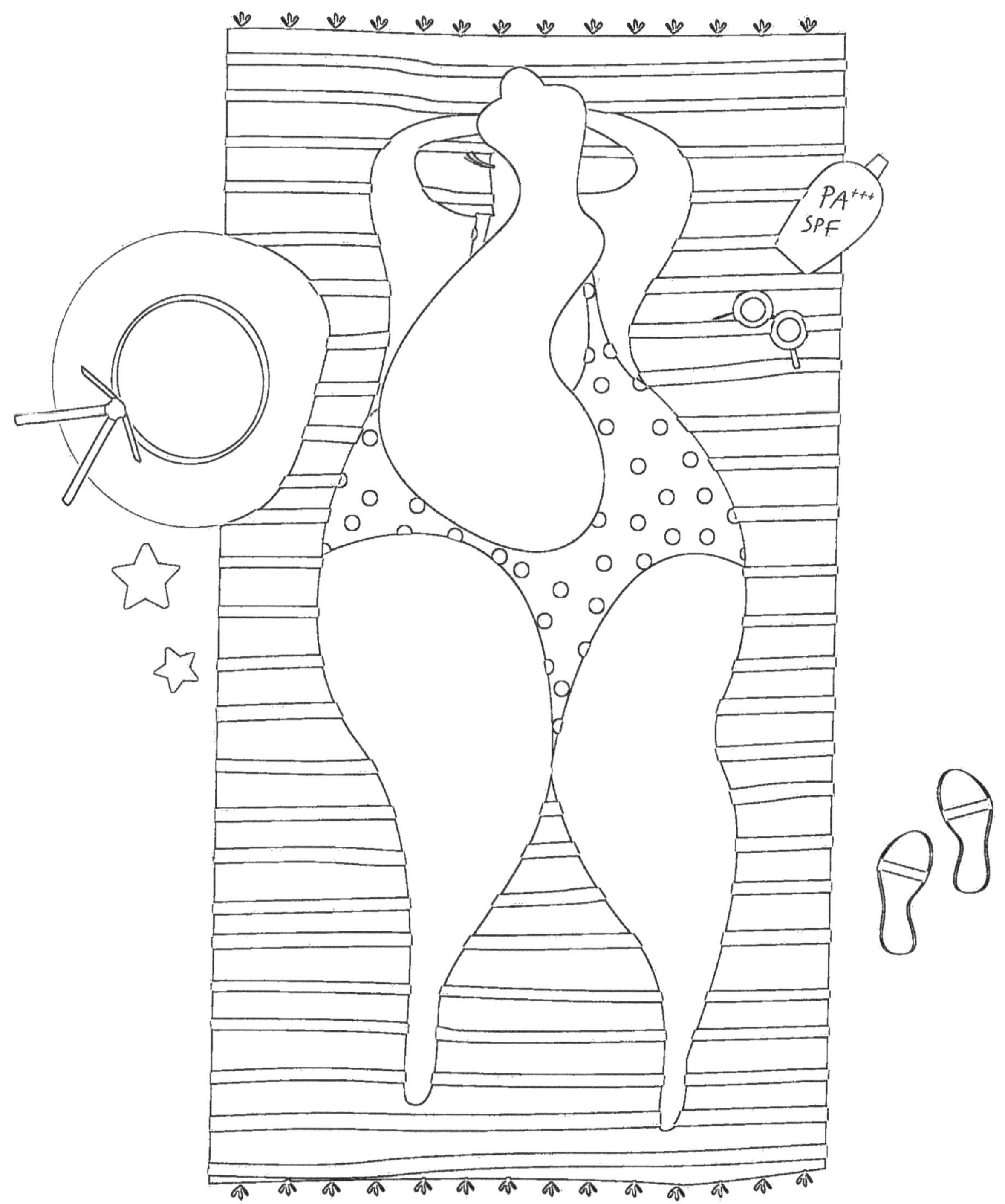
PA+++
SPF

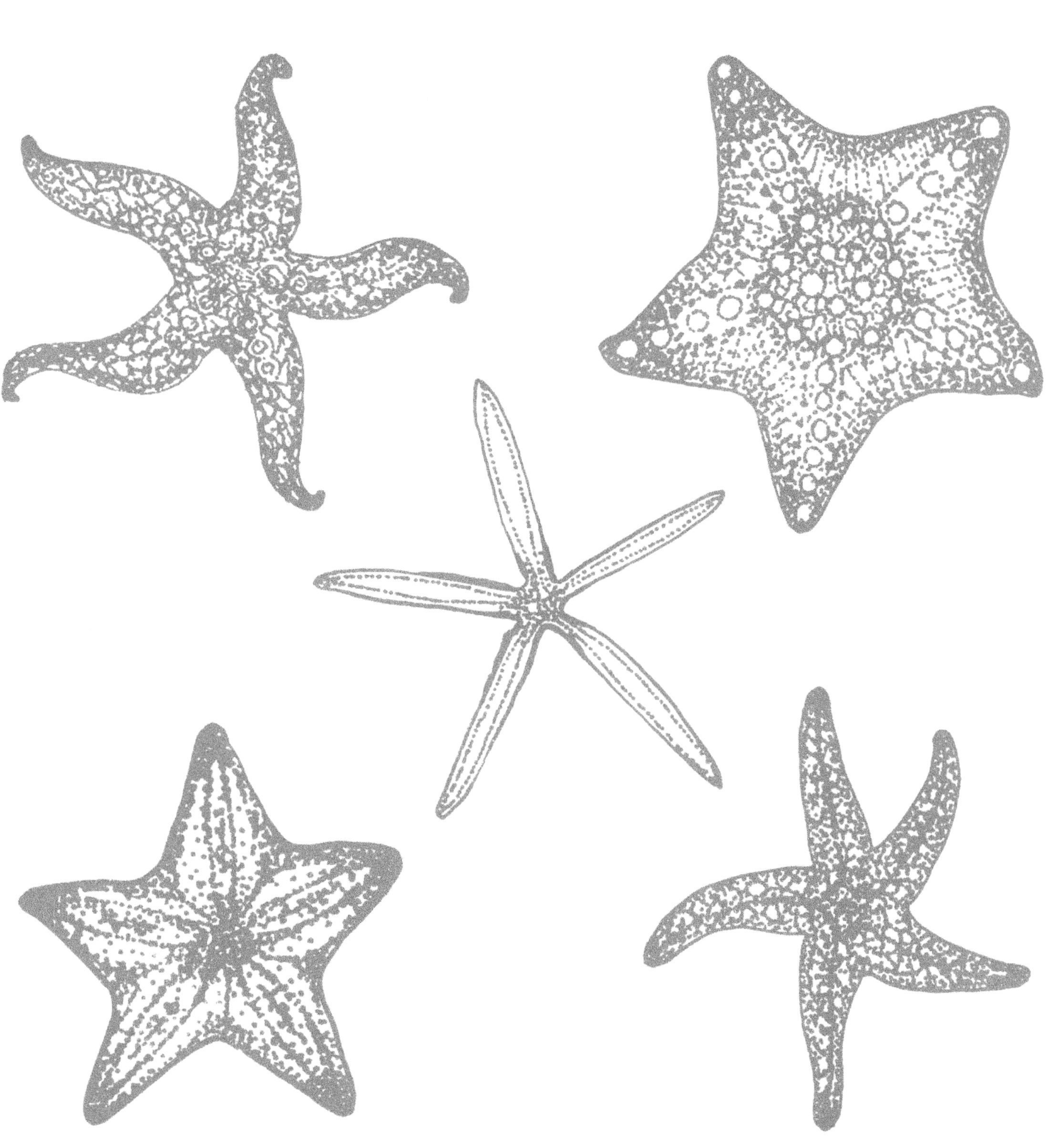

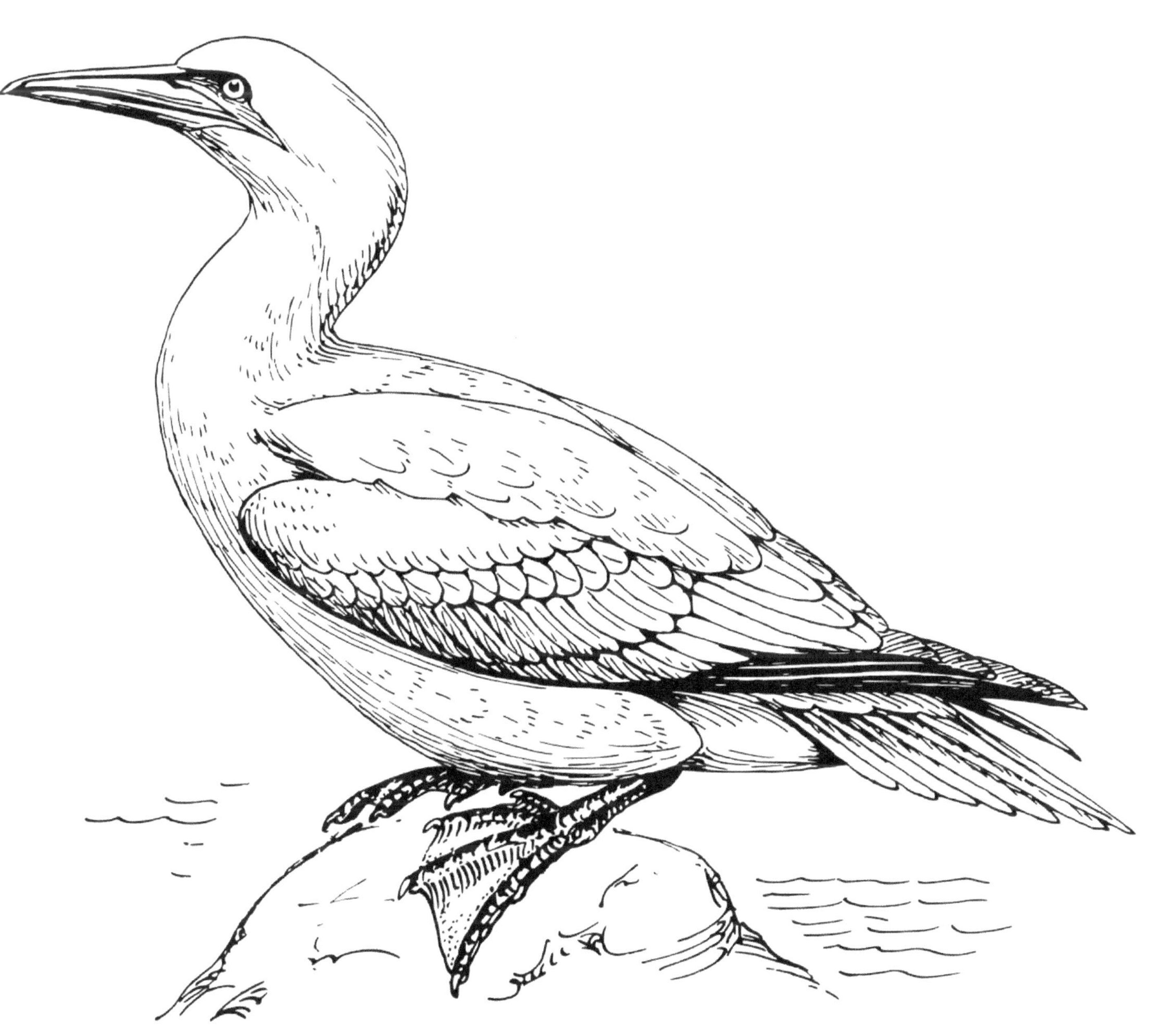

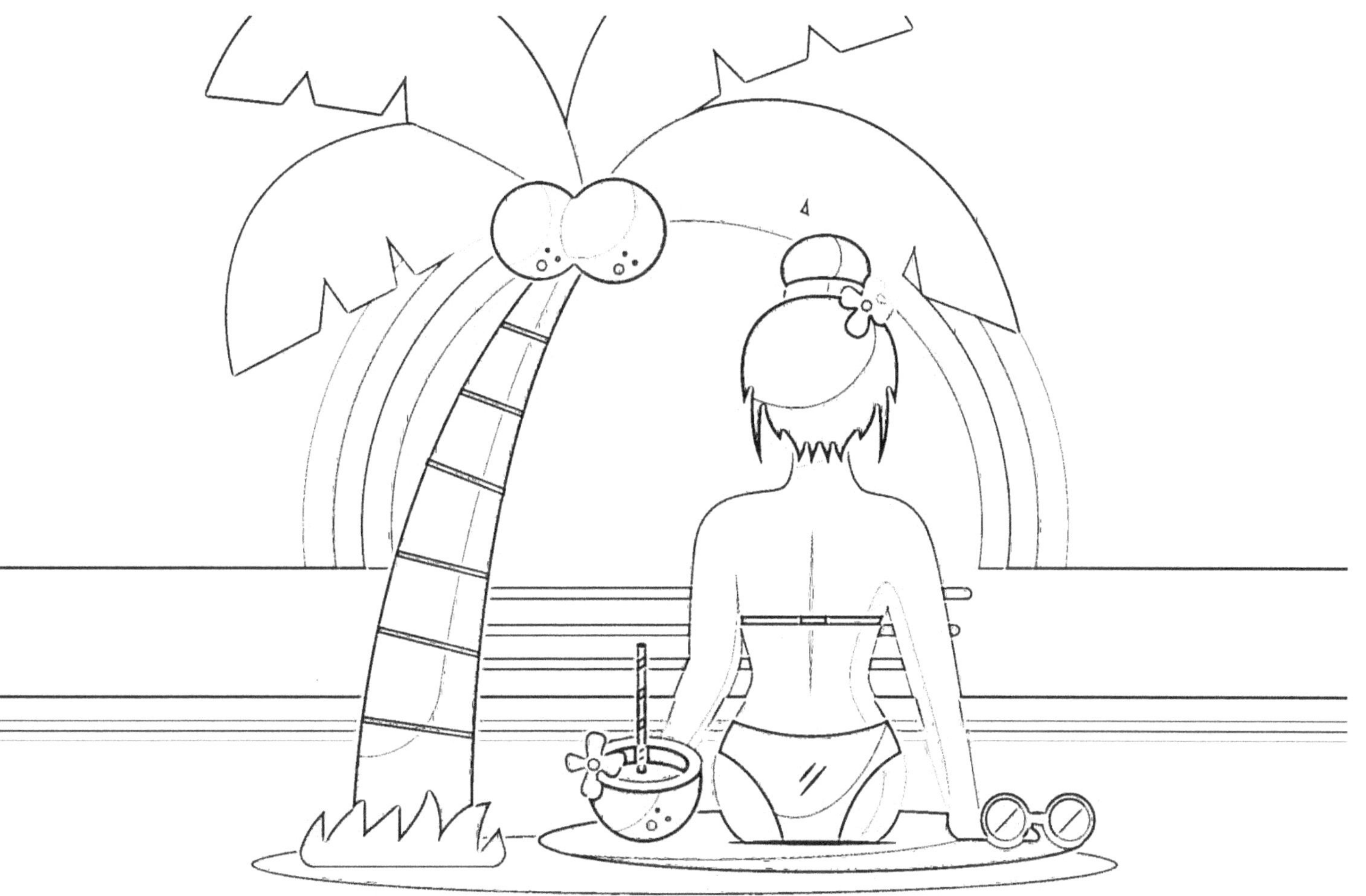

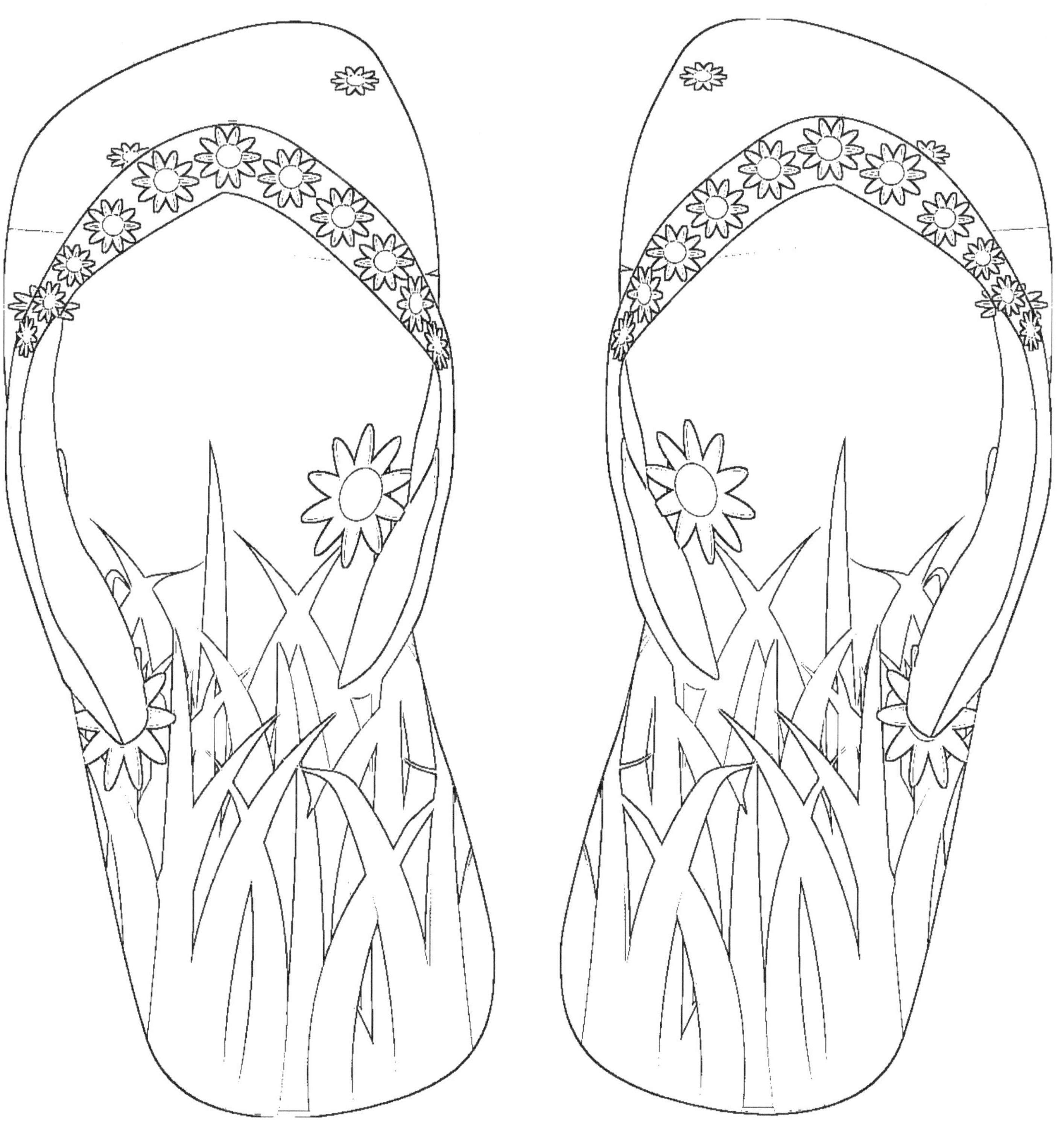

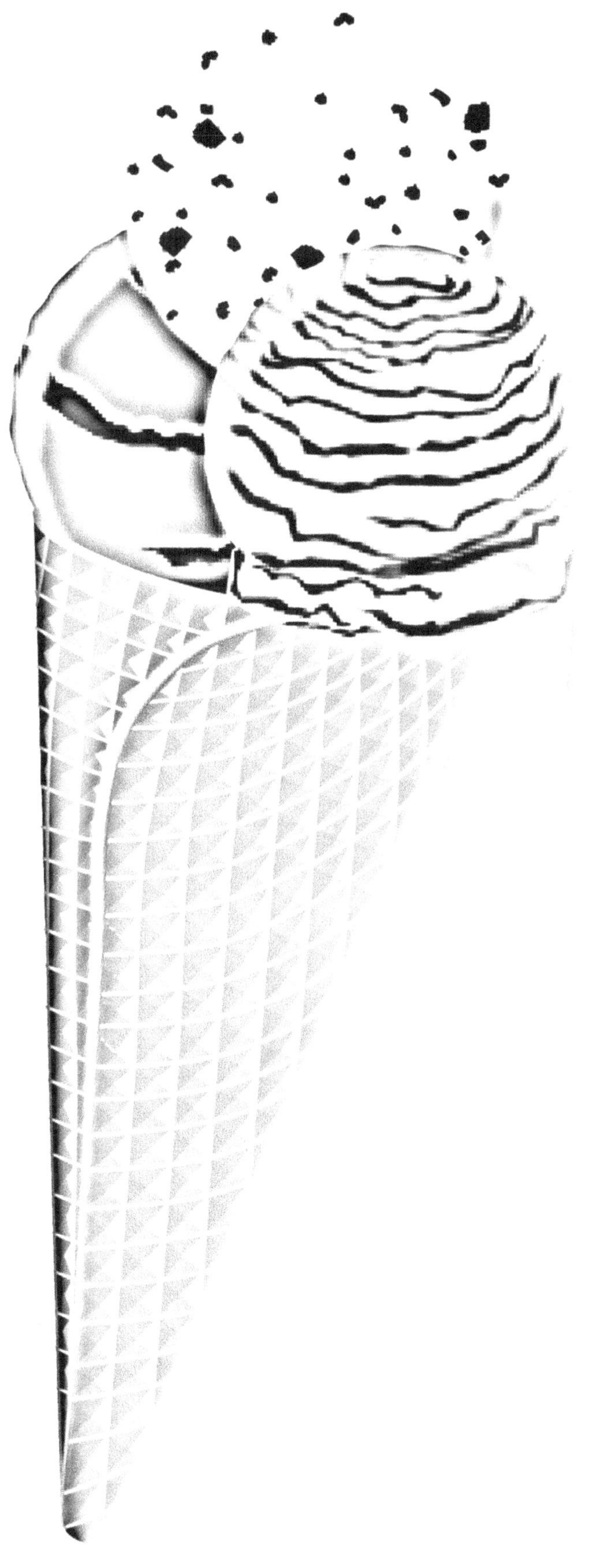

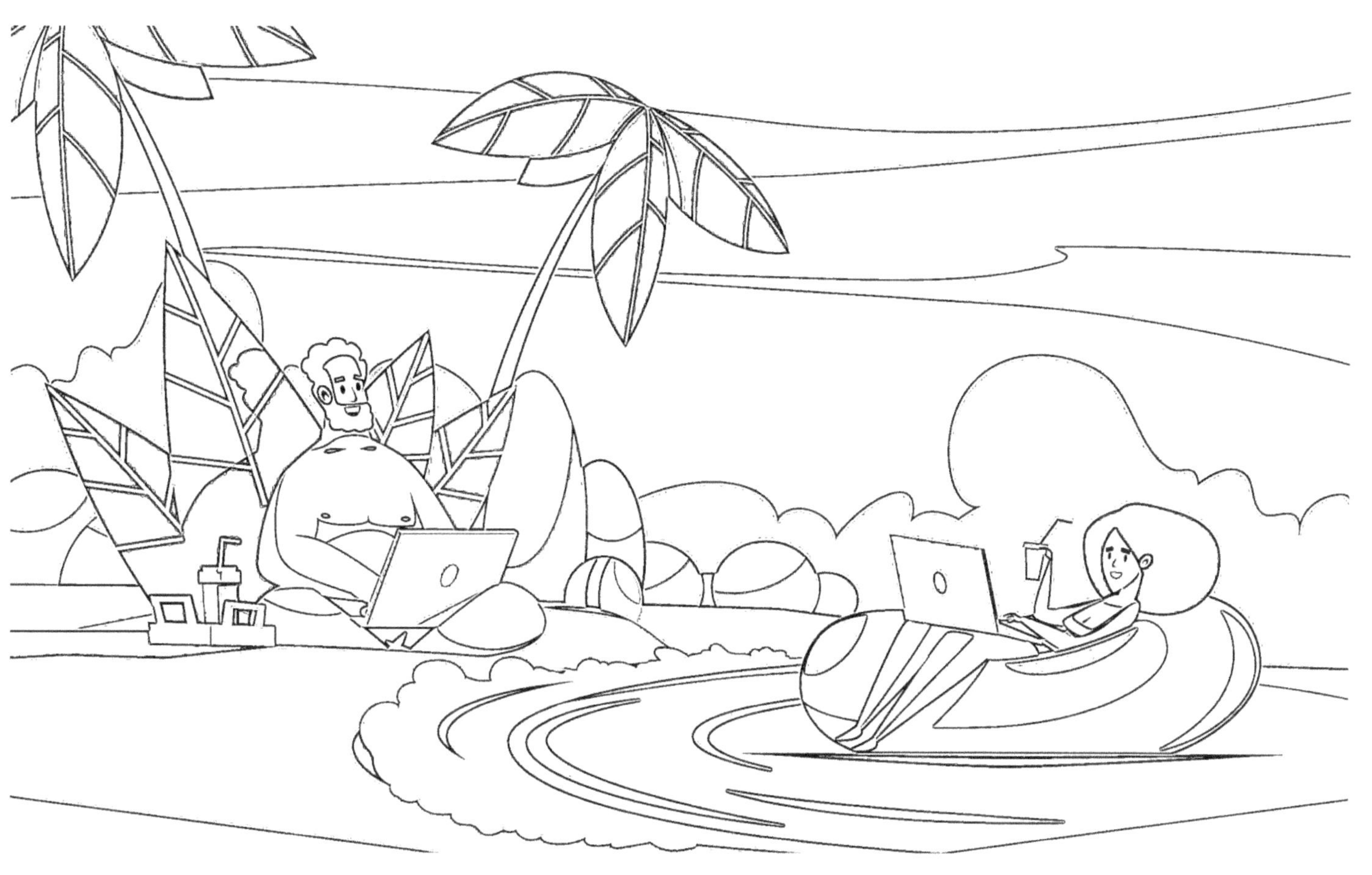

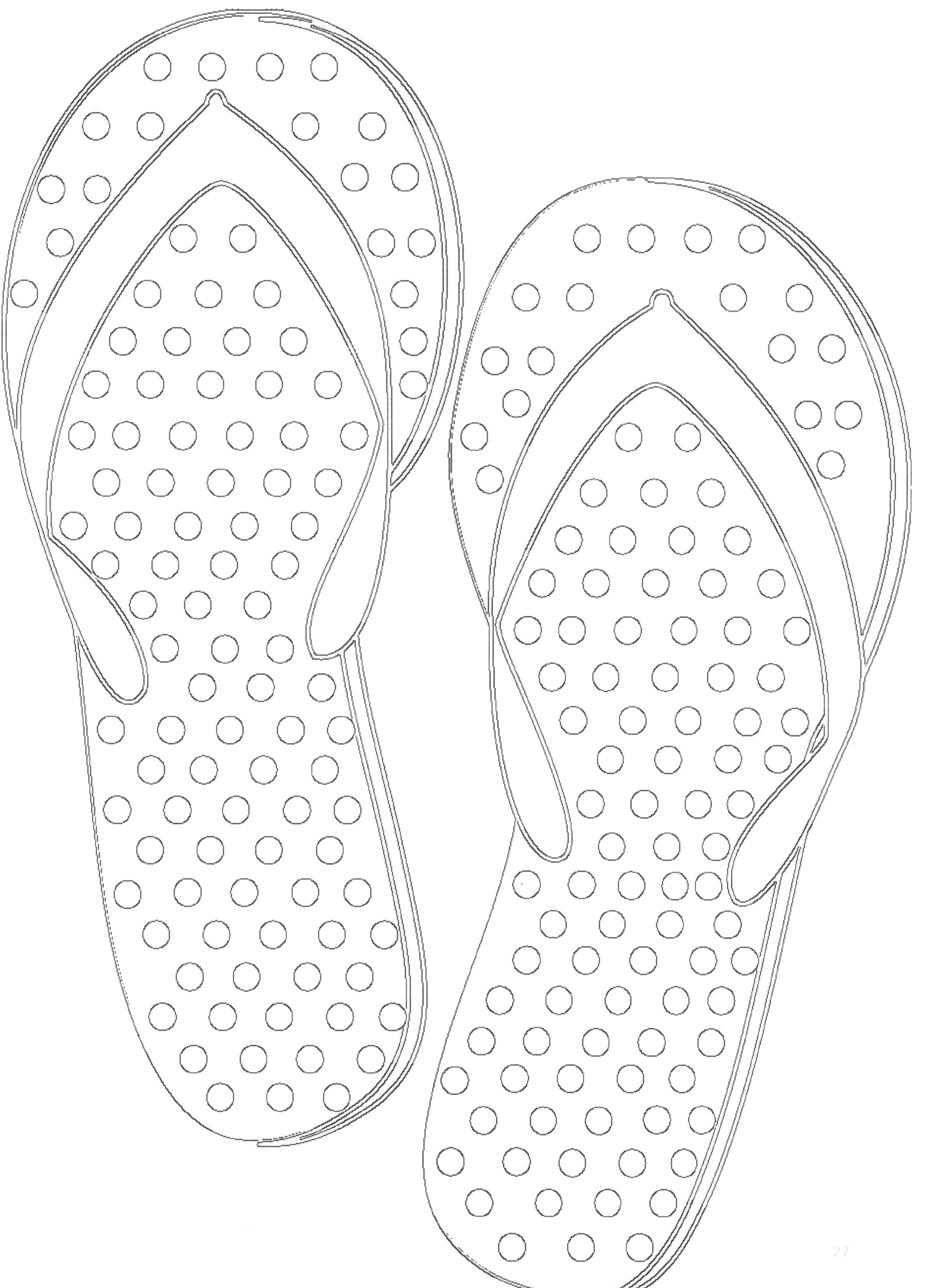

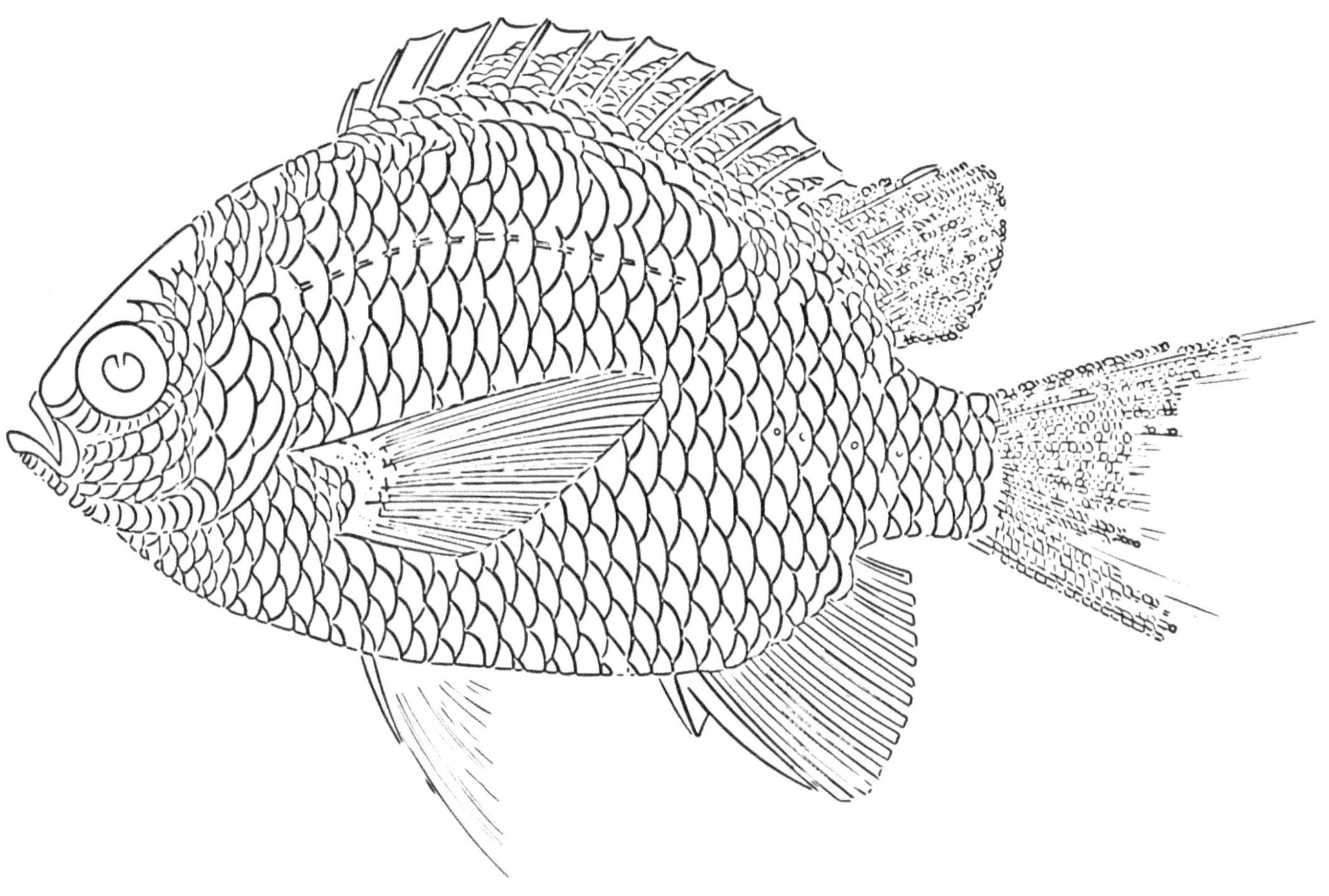

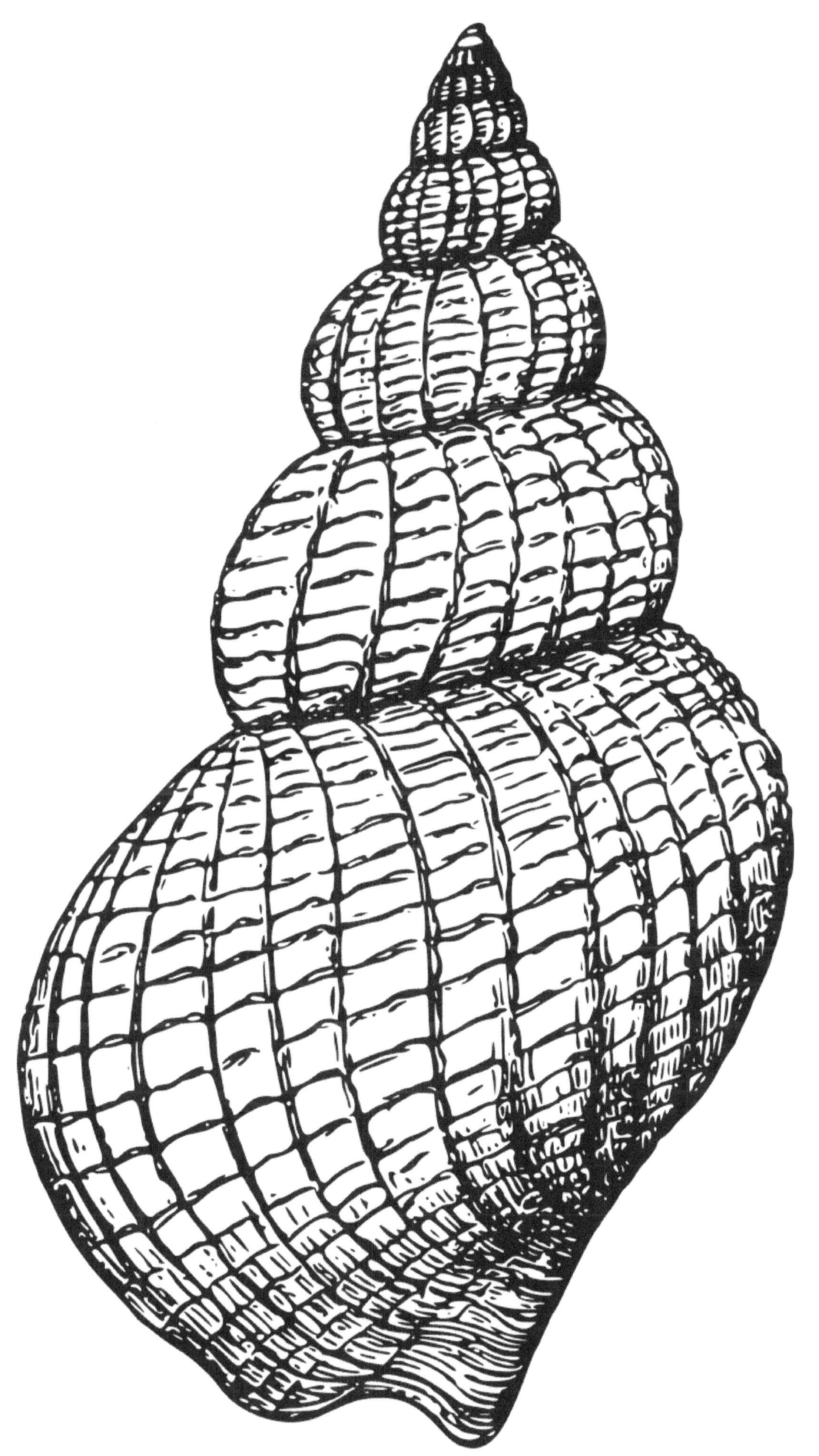

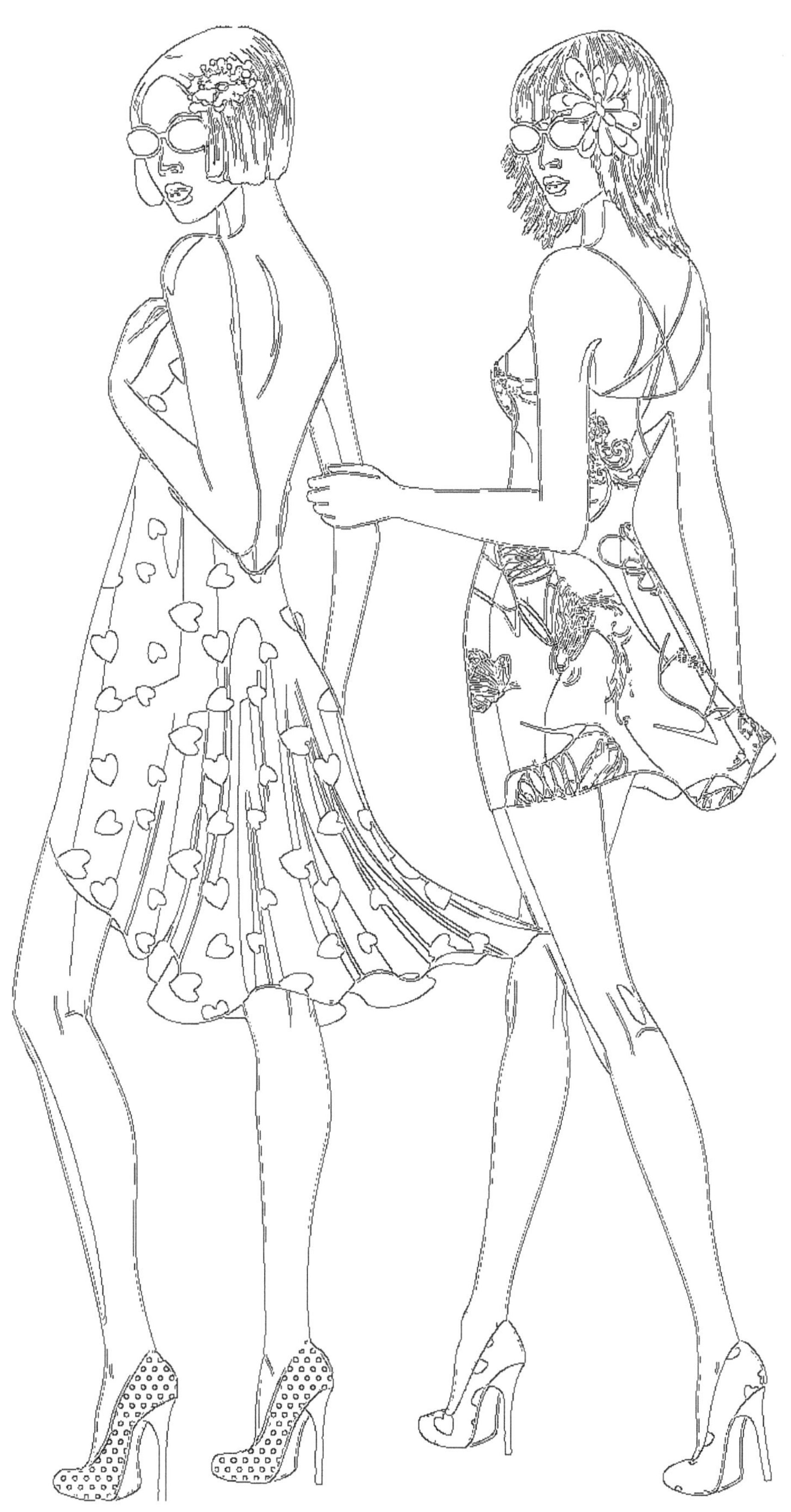

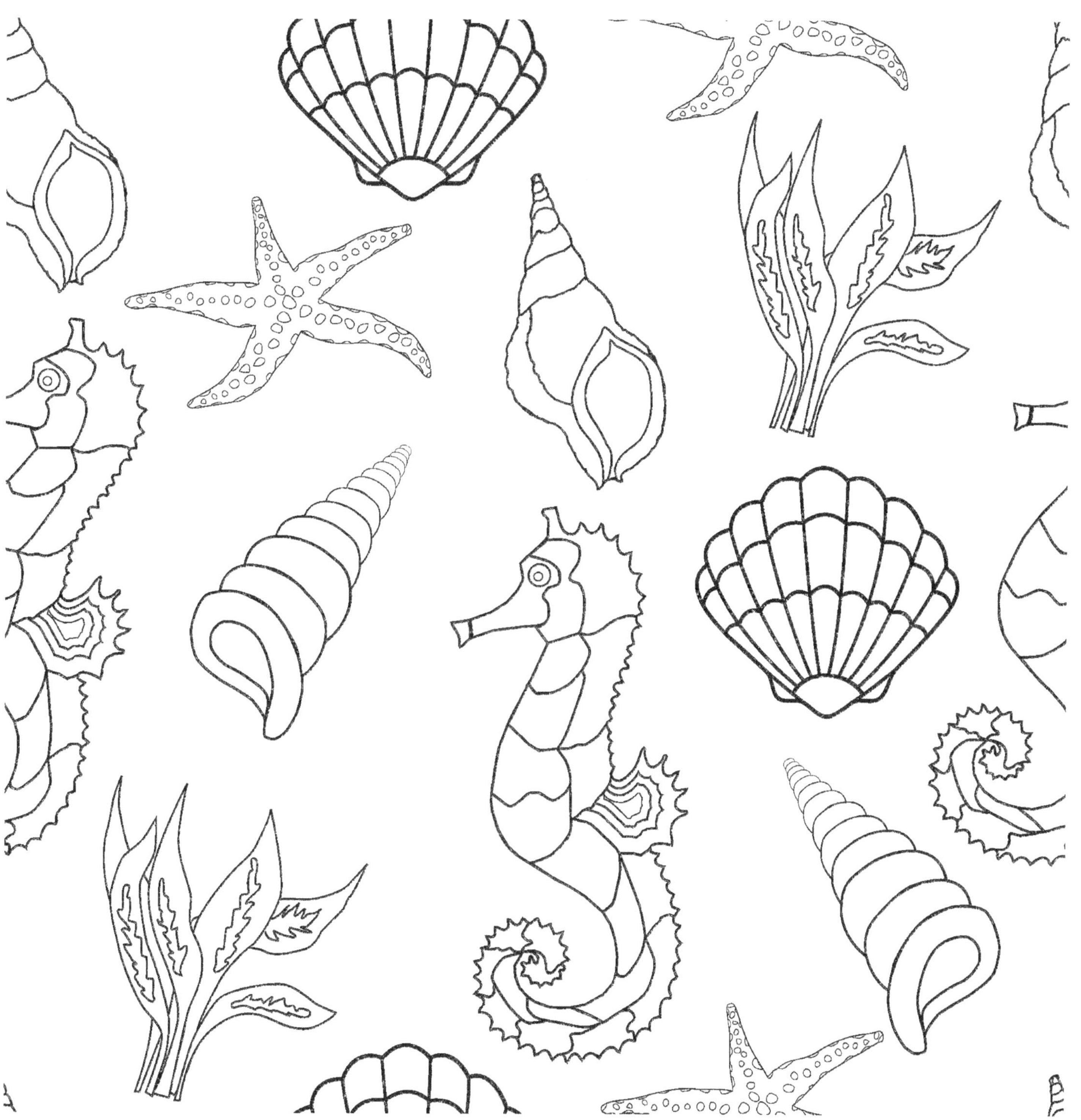

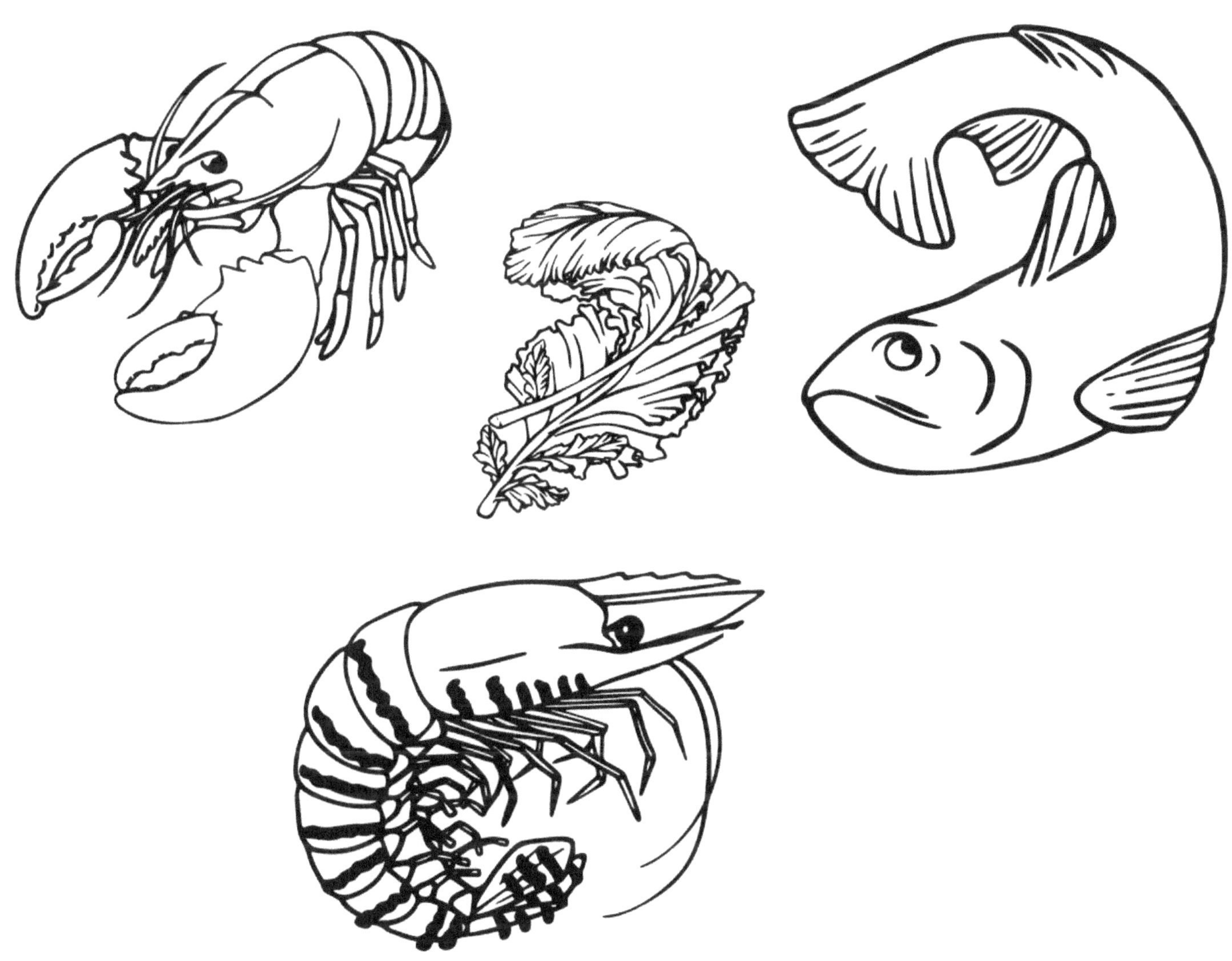

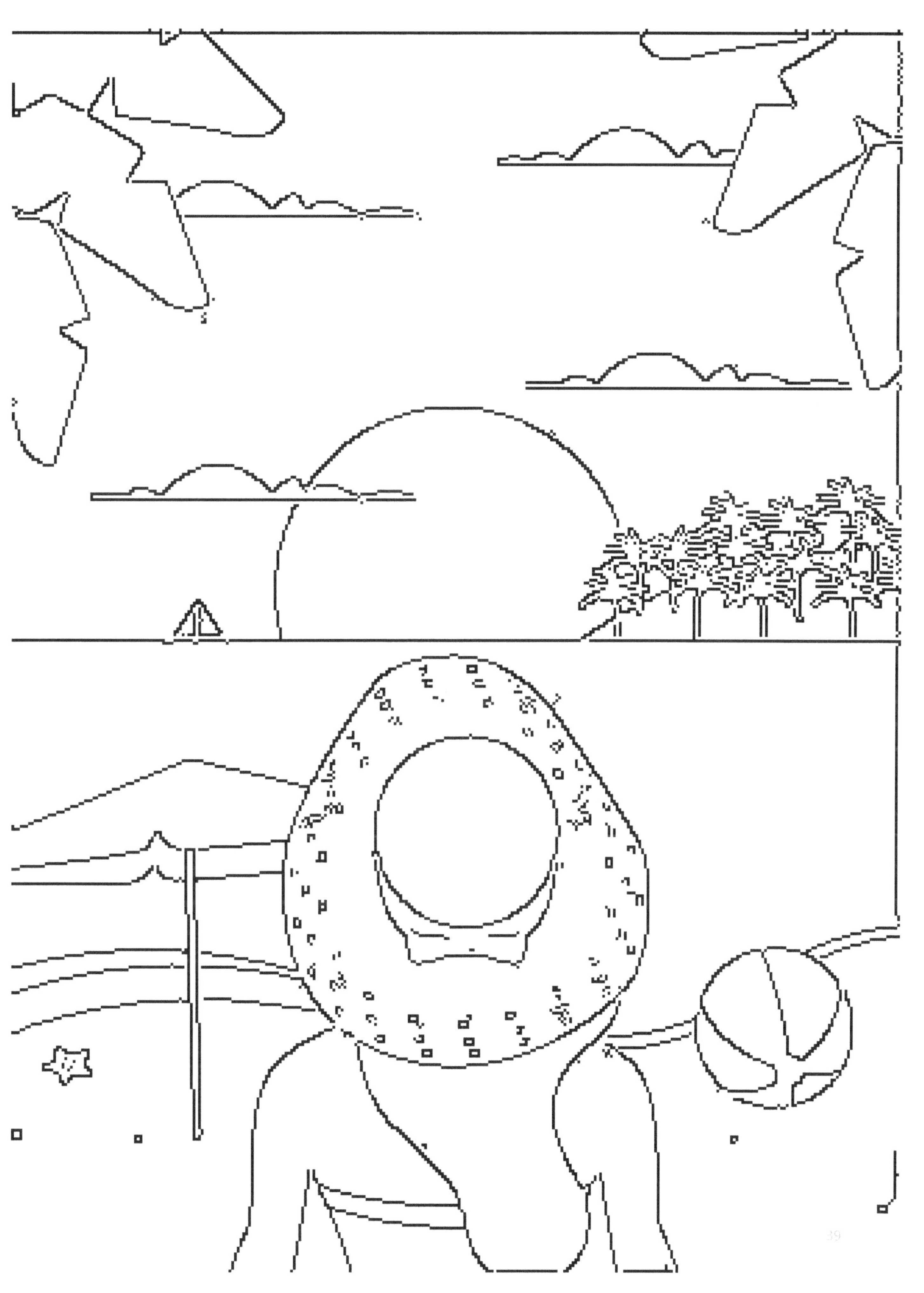

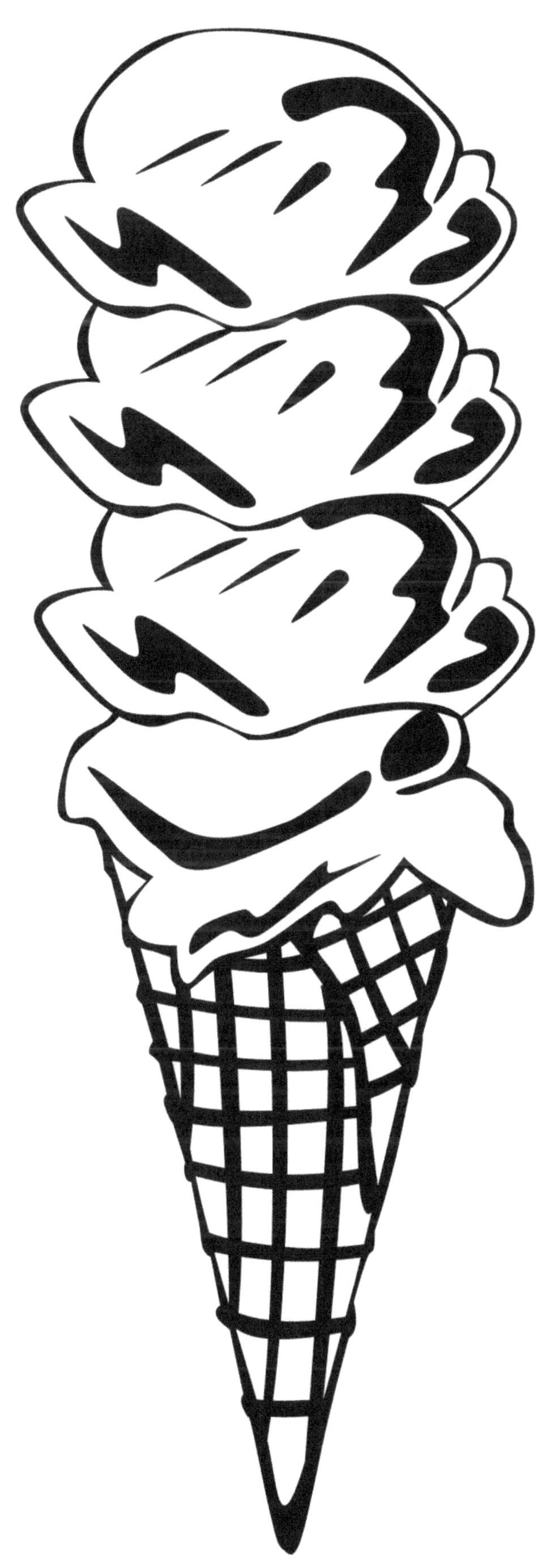

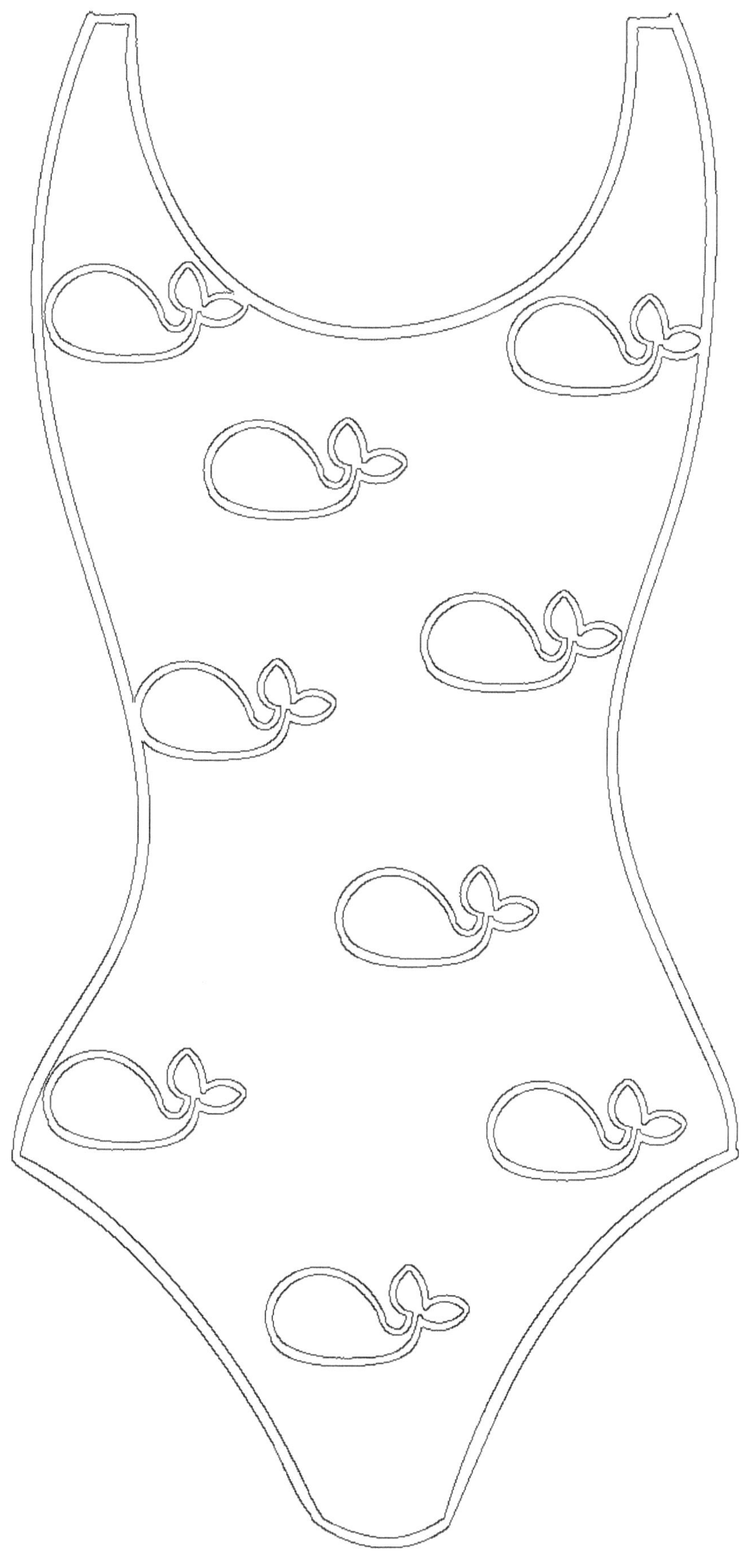

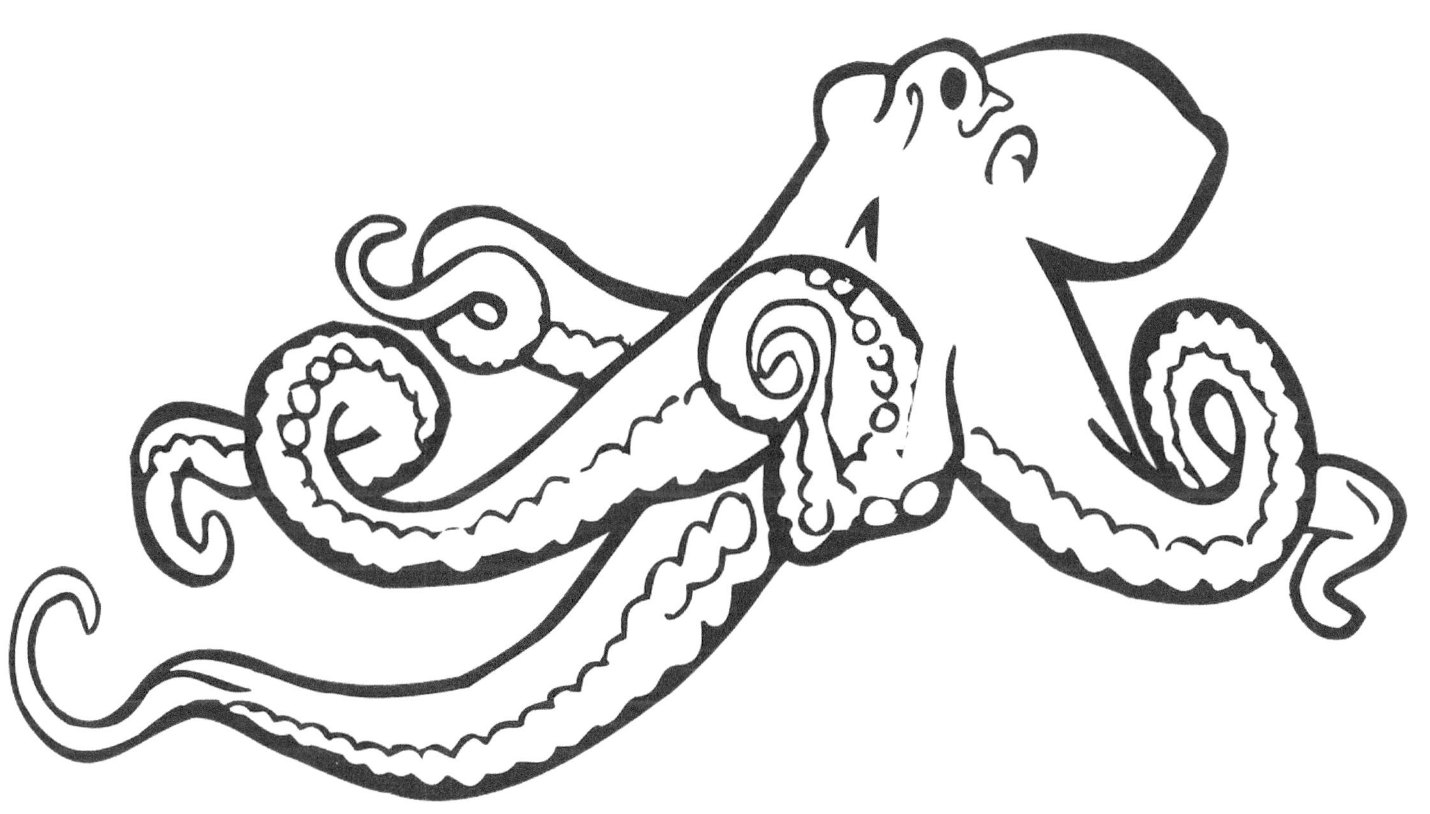

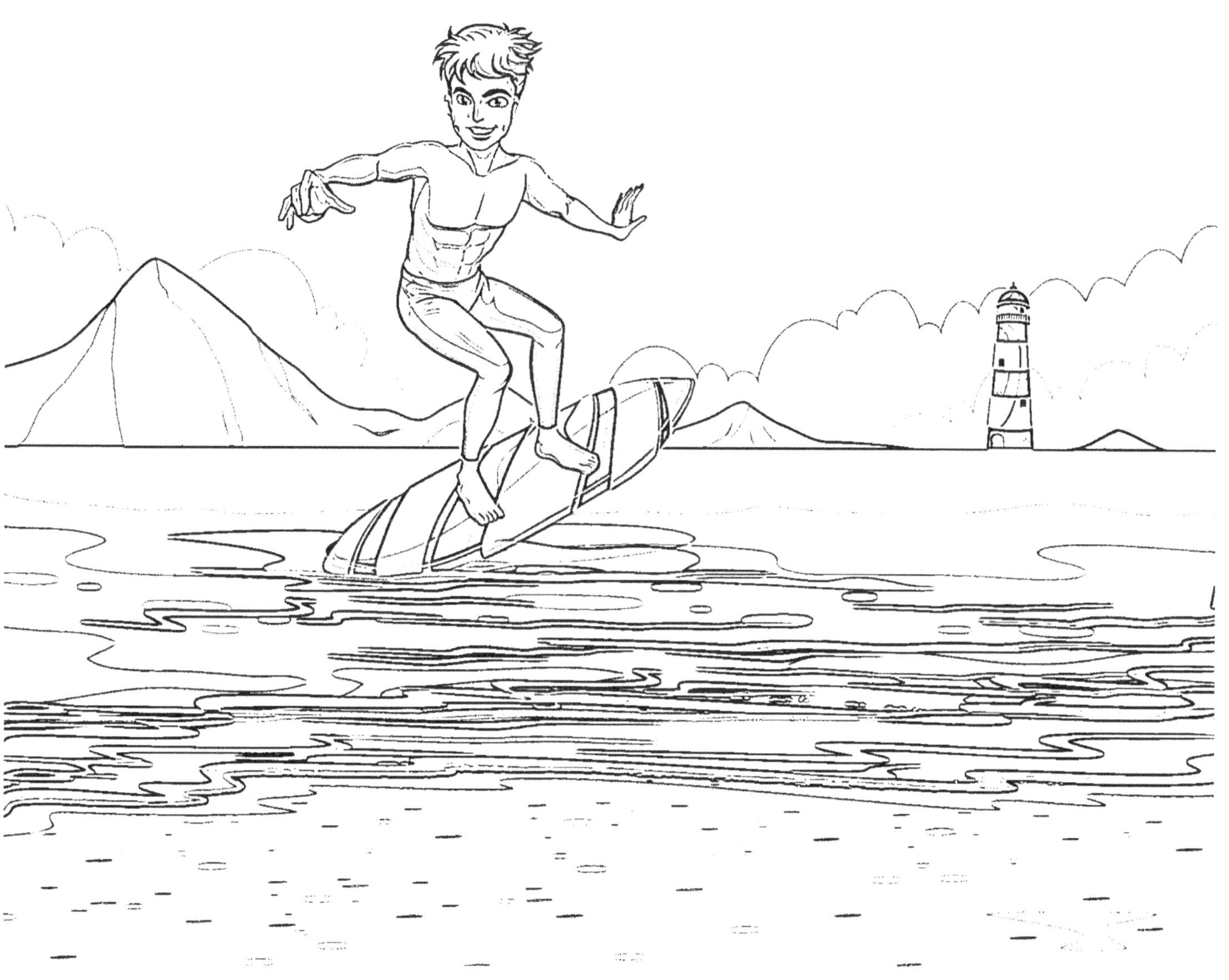

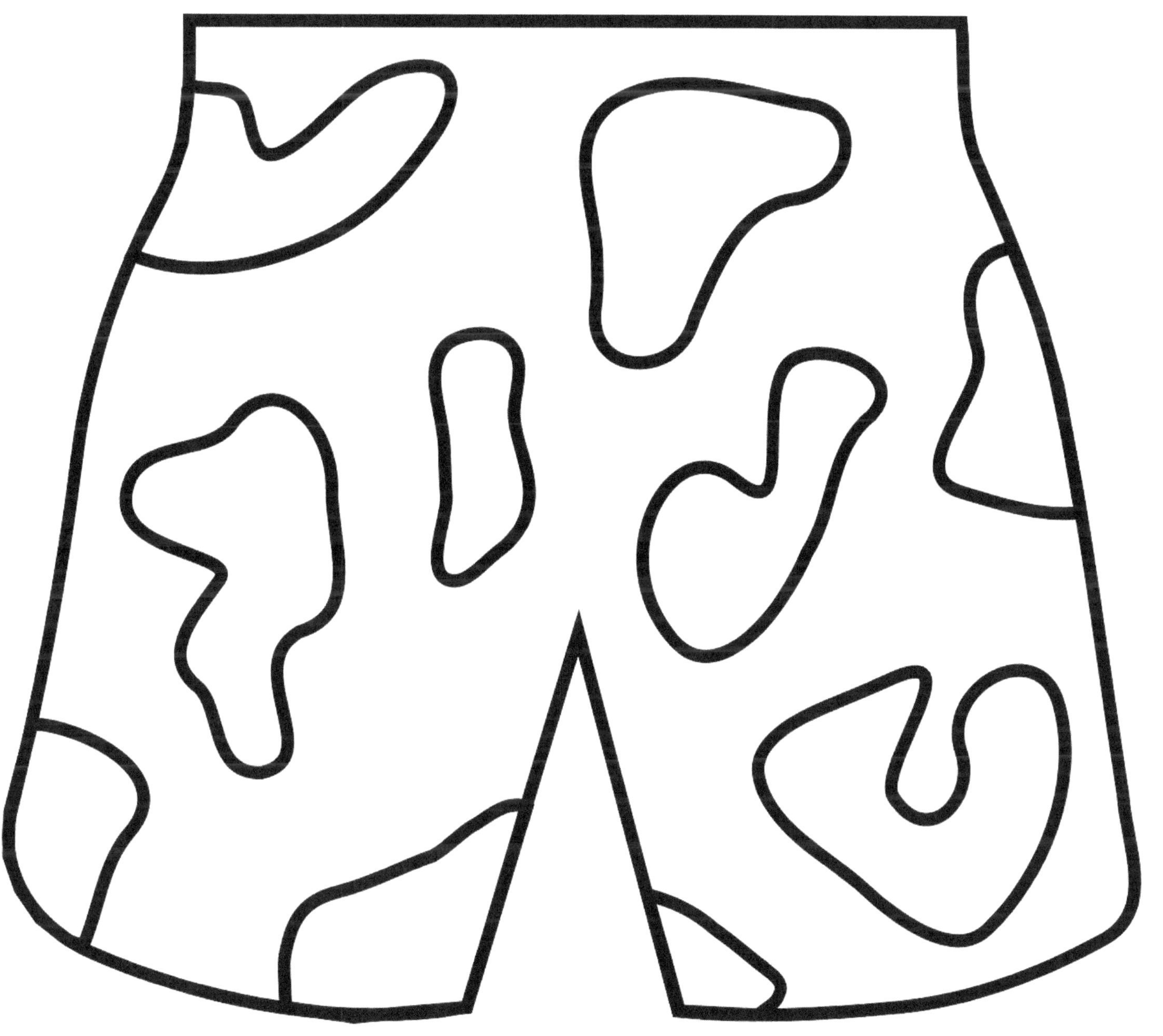

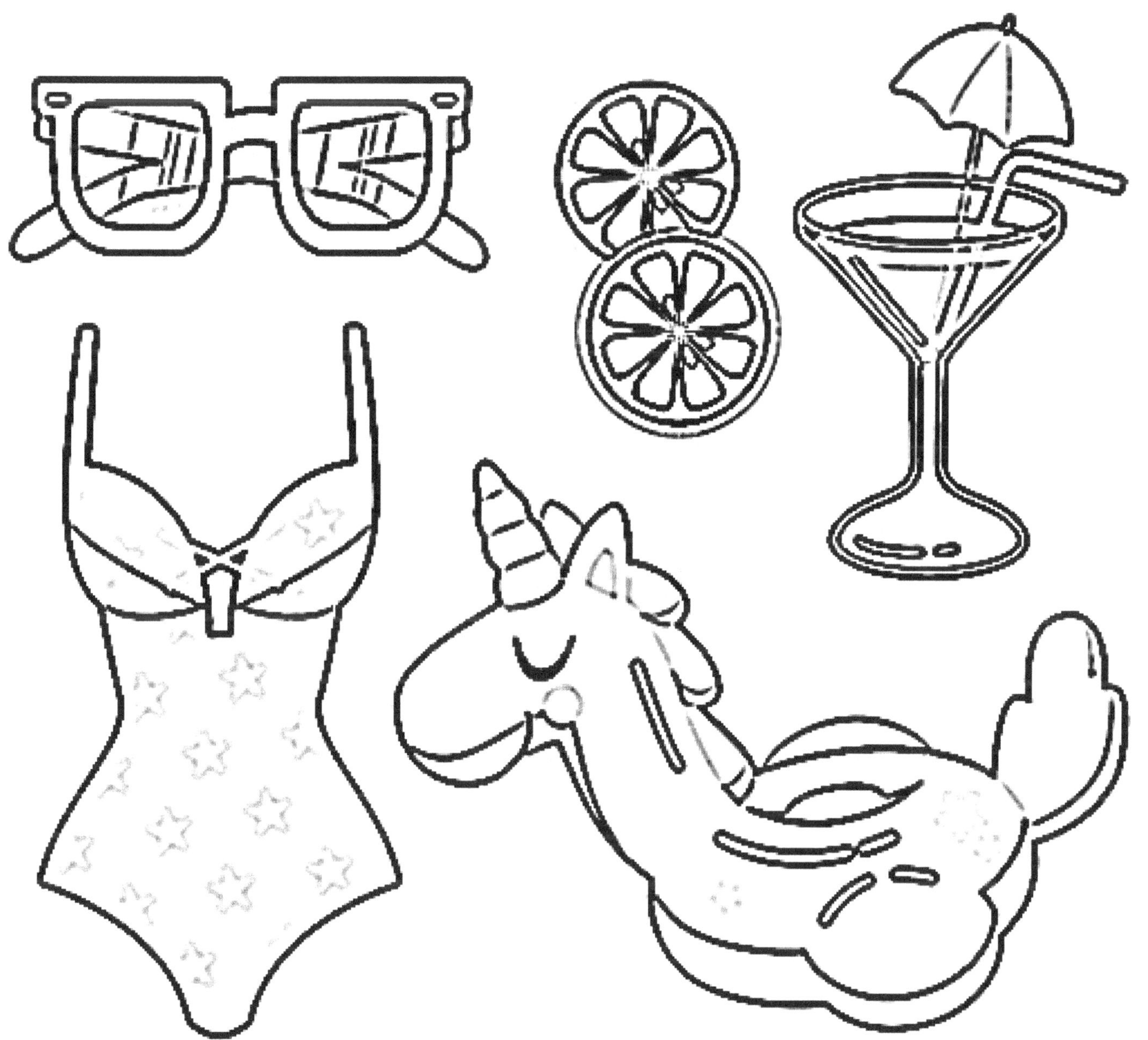

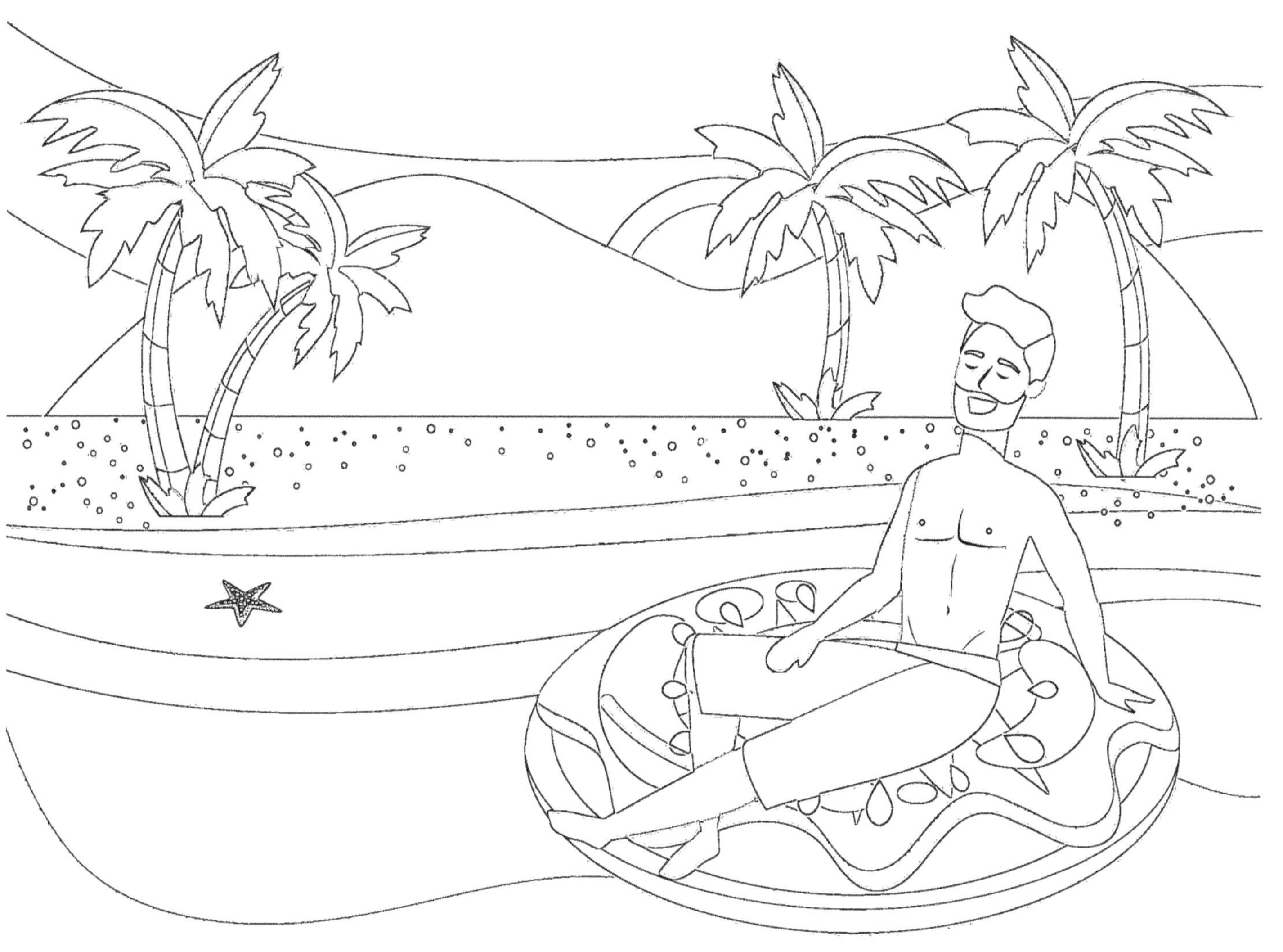

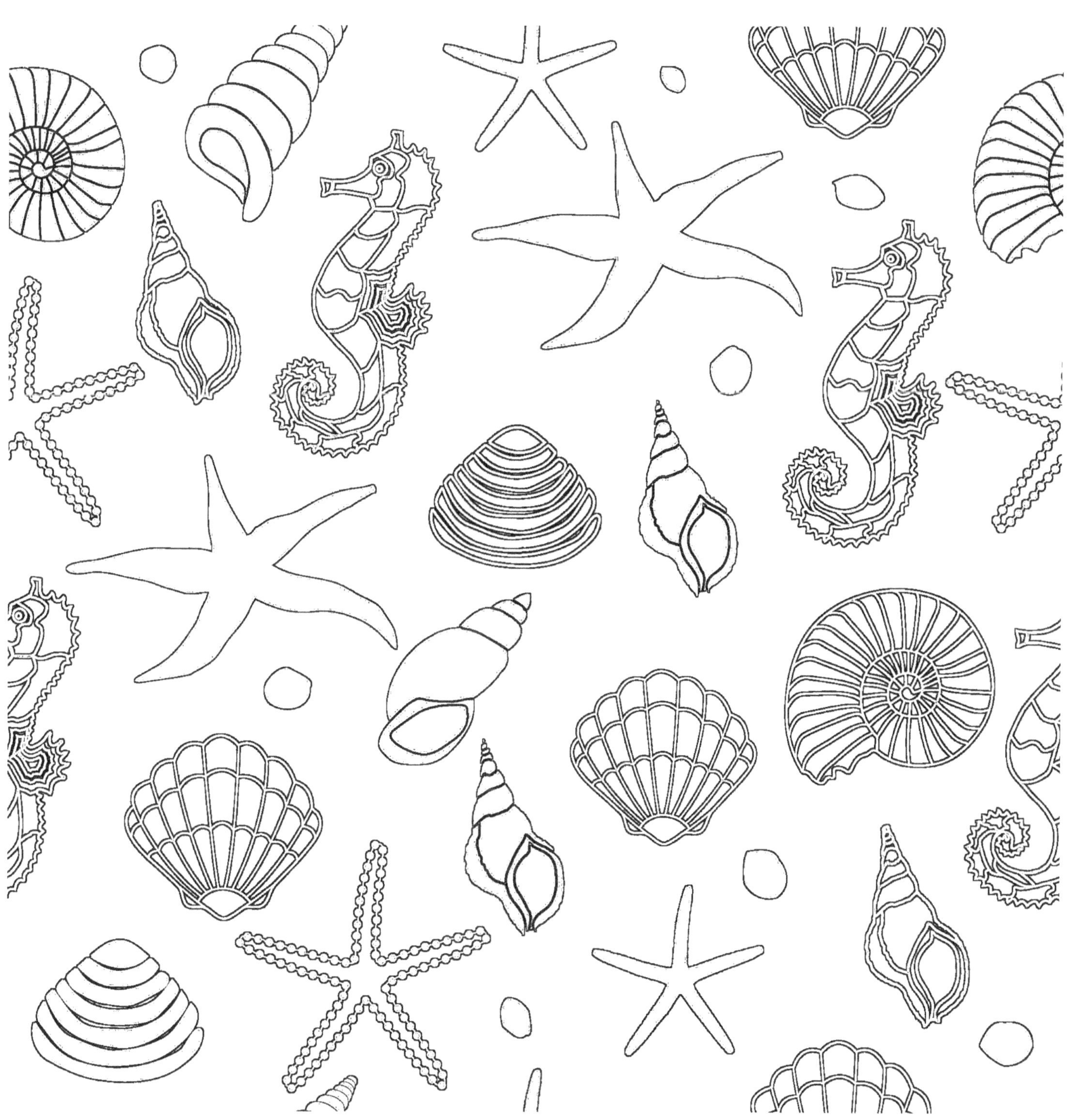

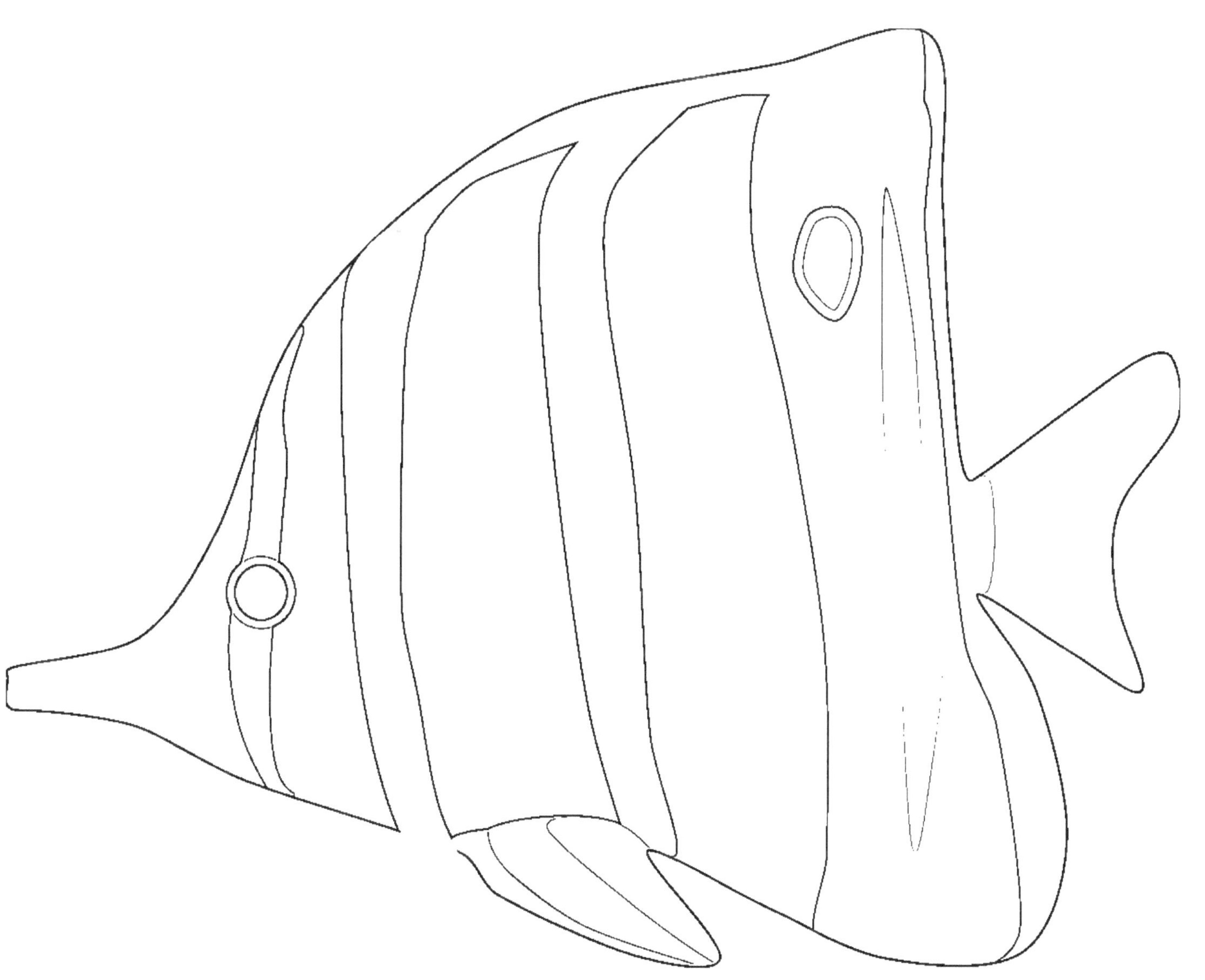

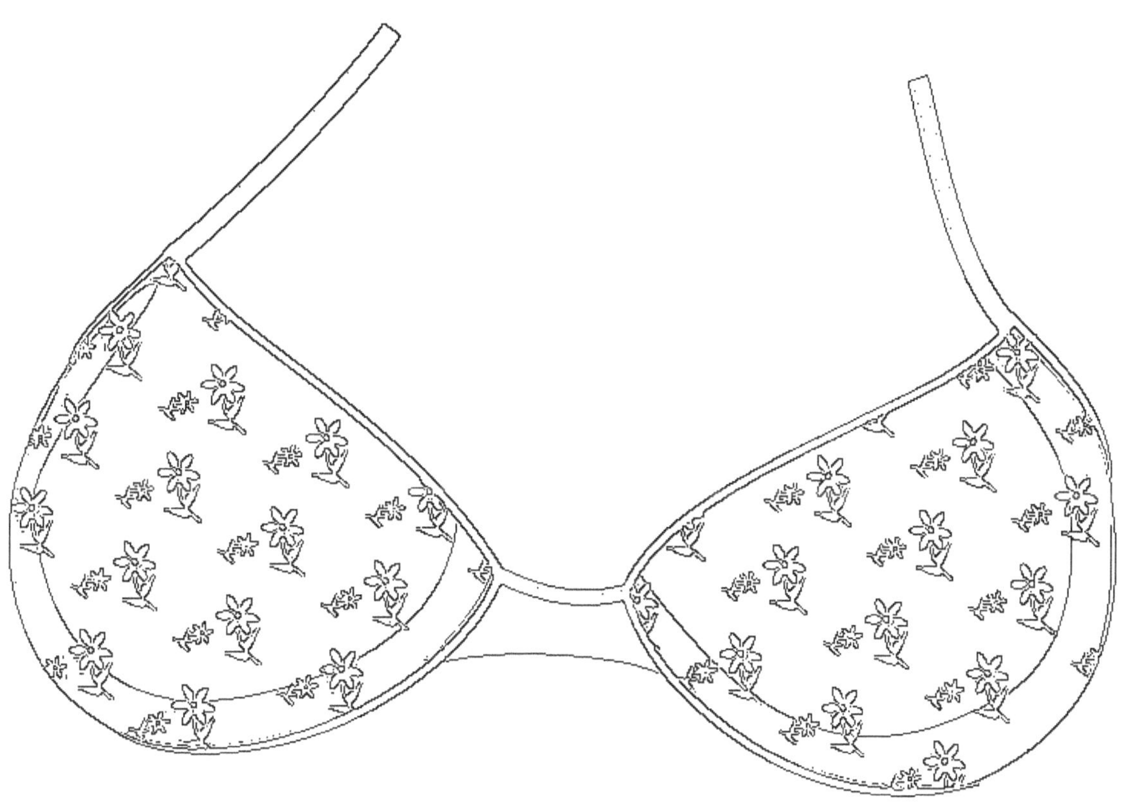

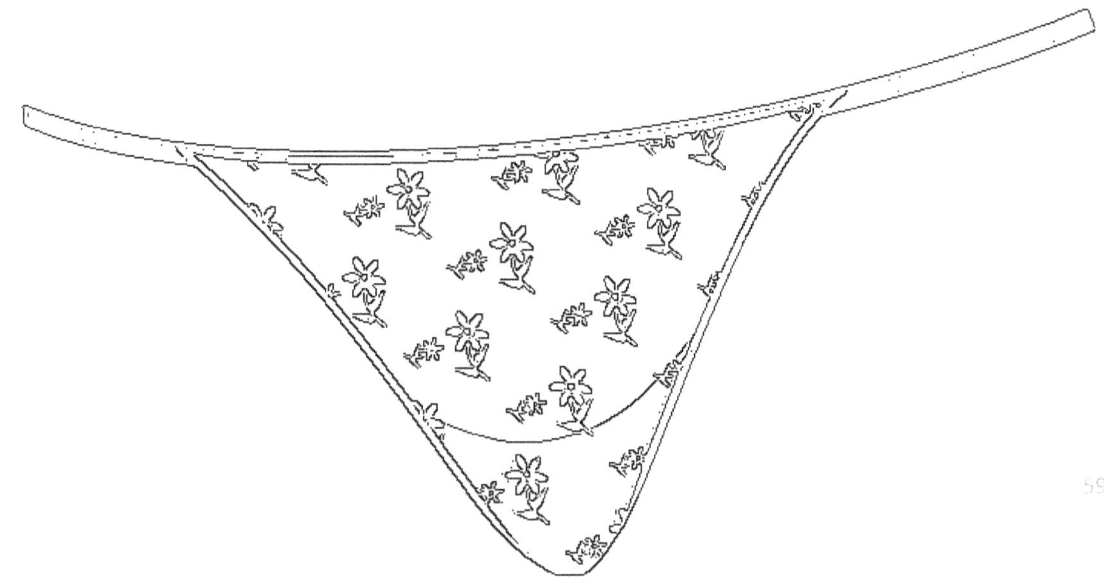

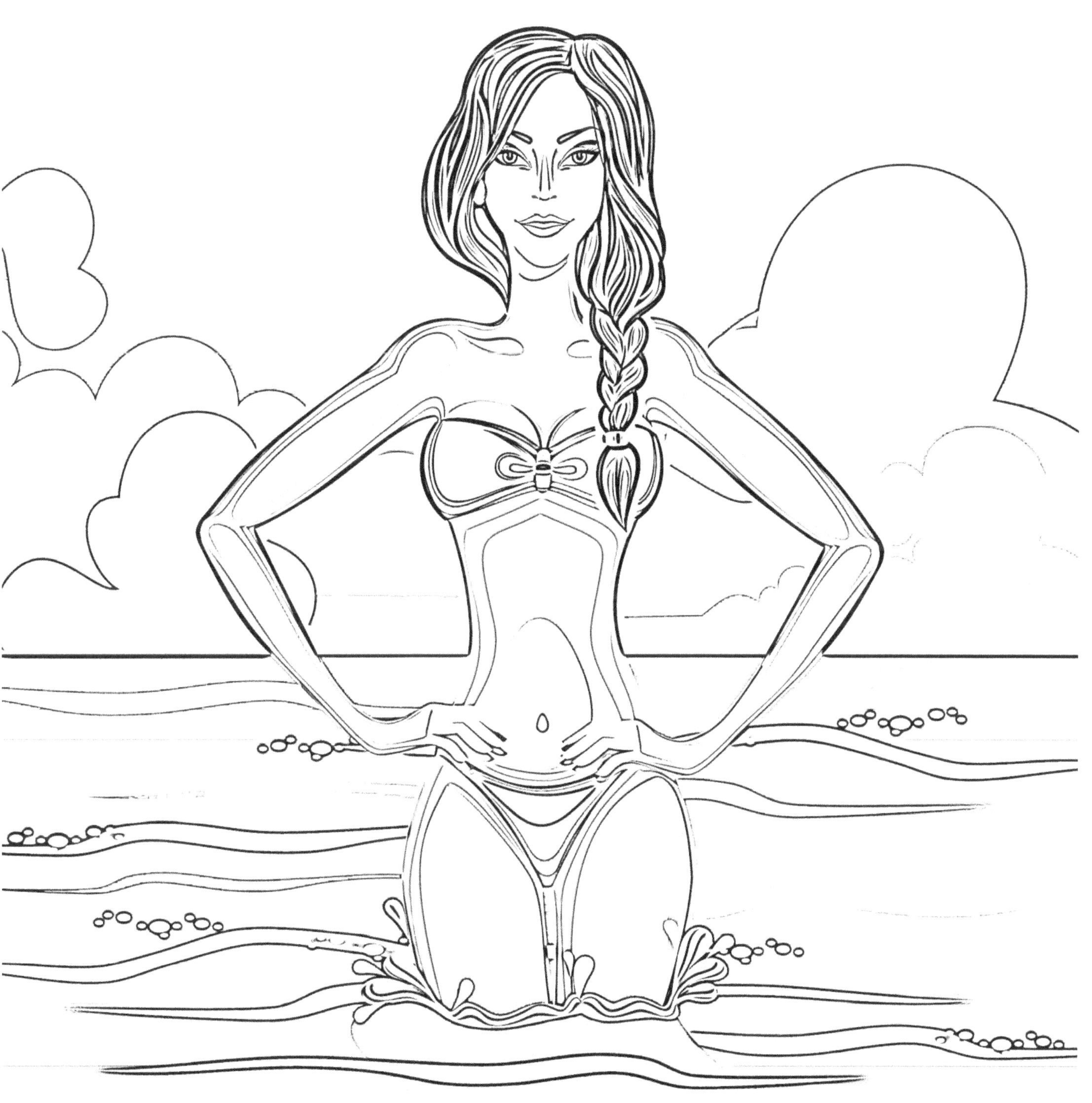

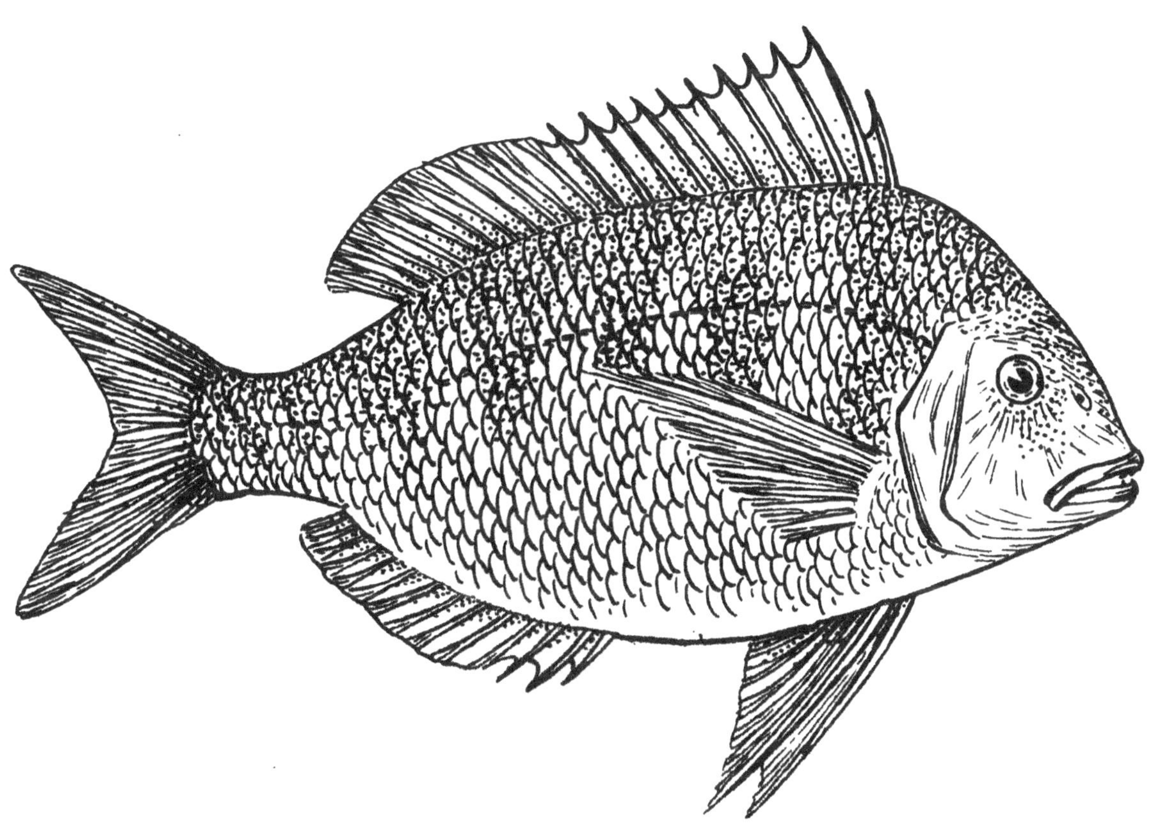

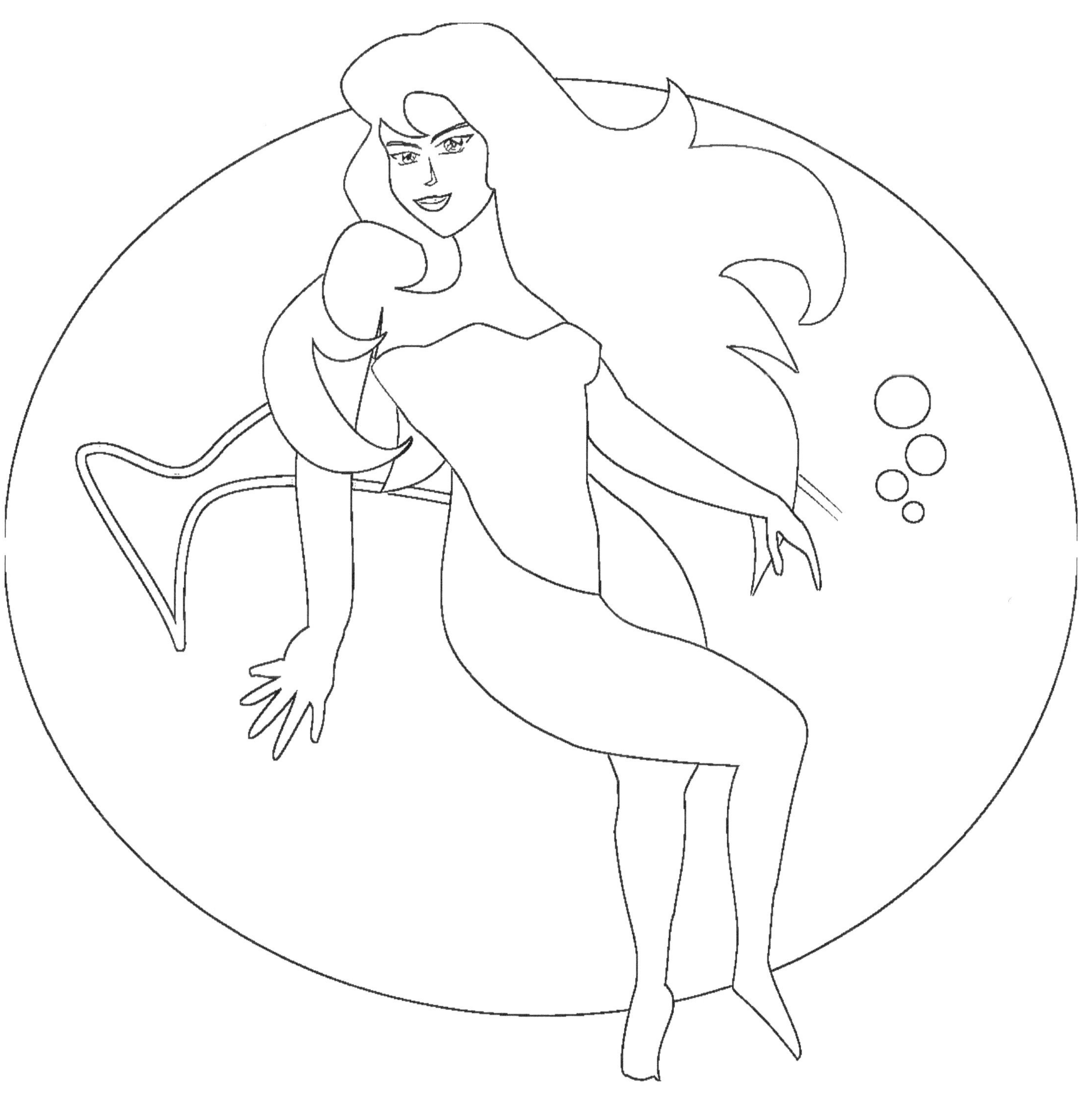

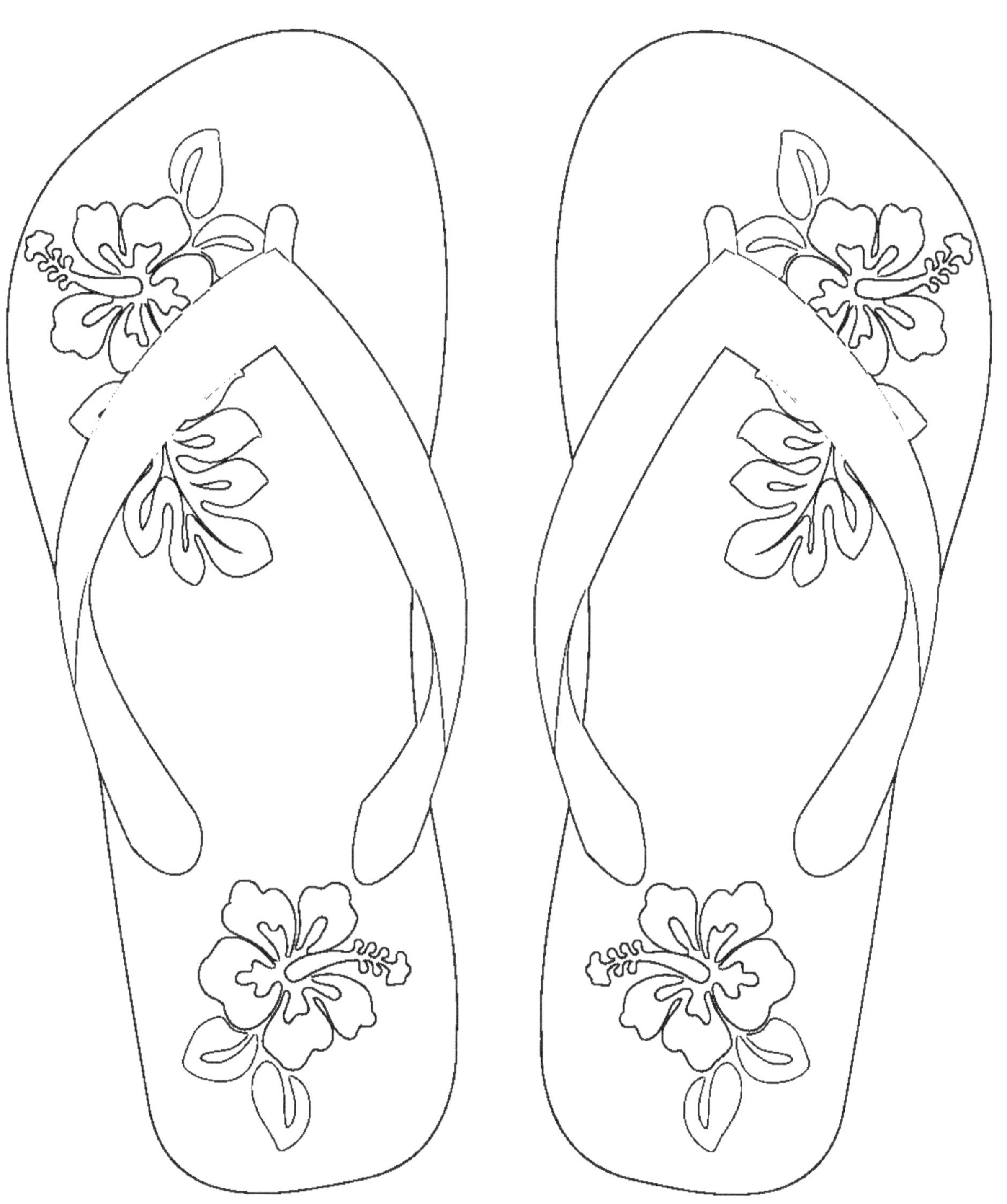

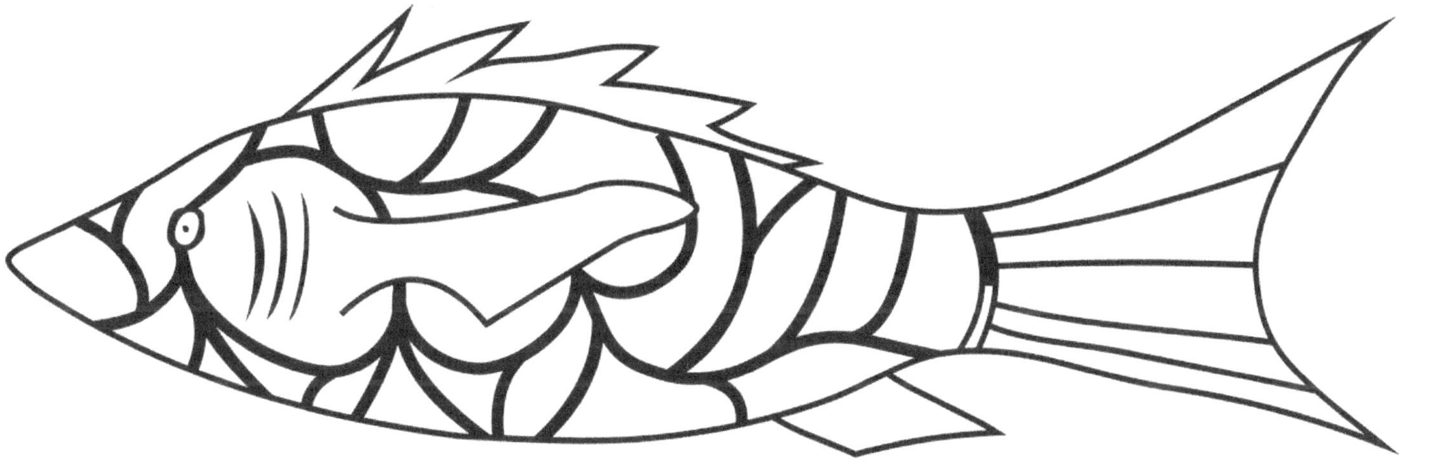

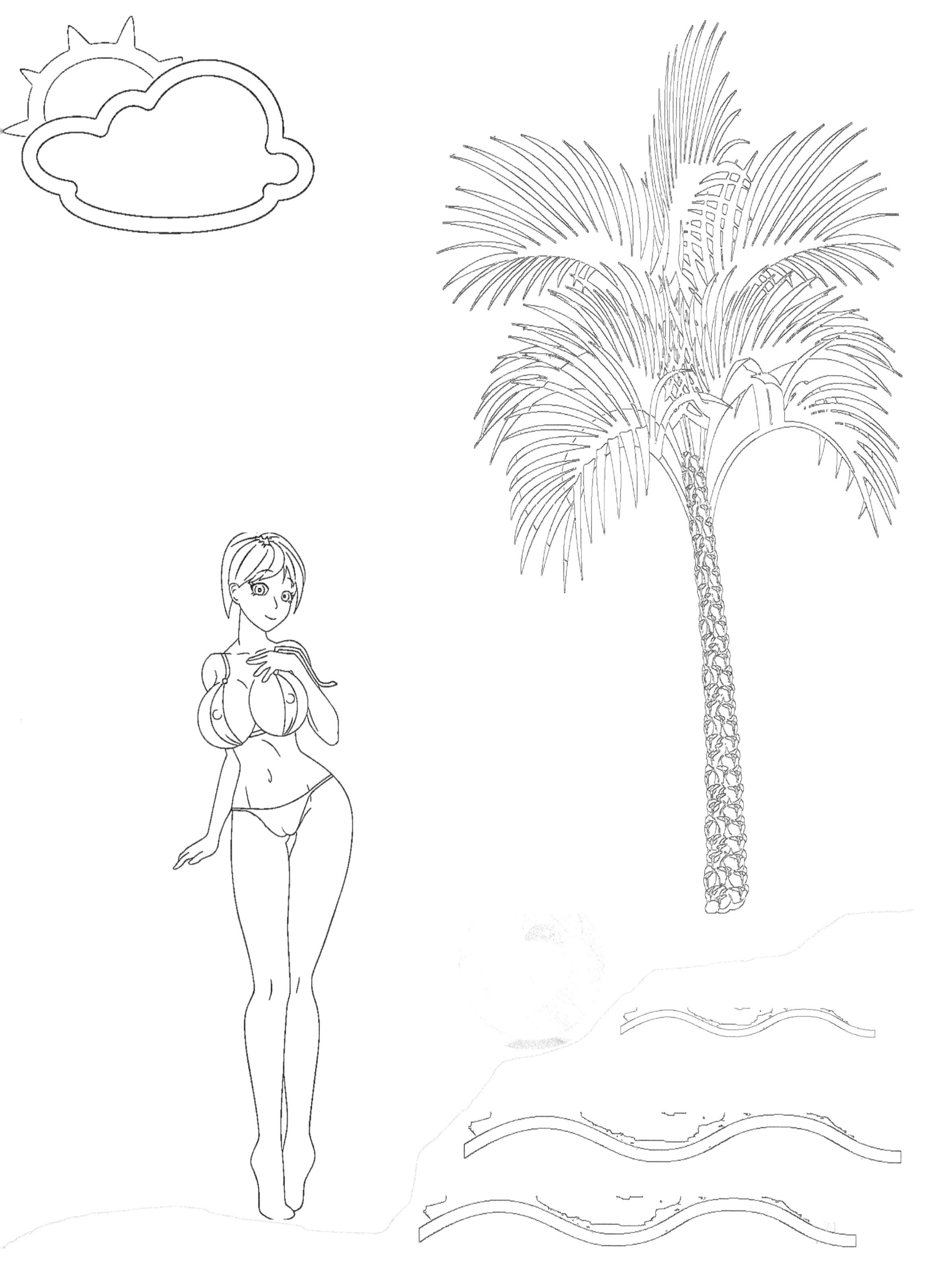

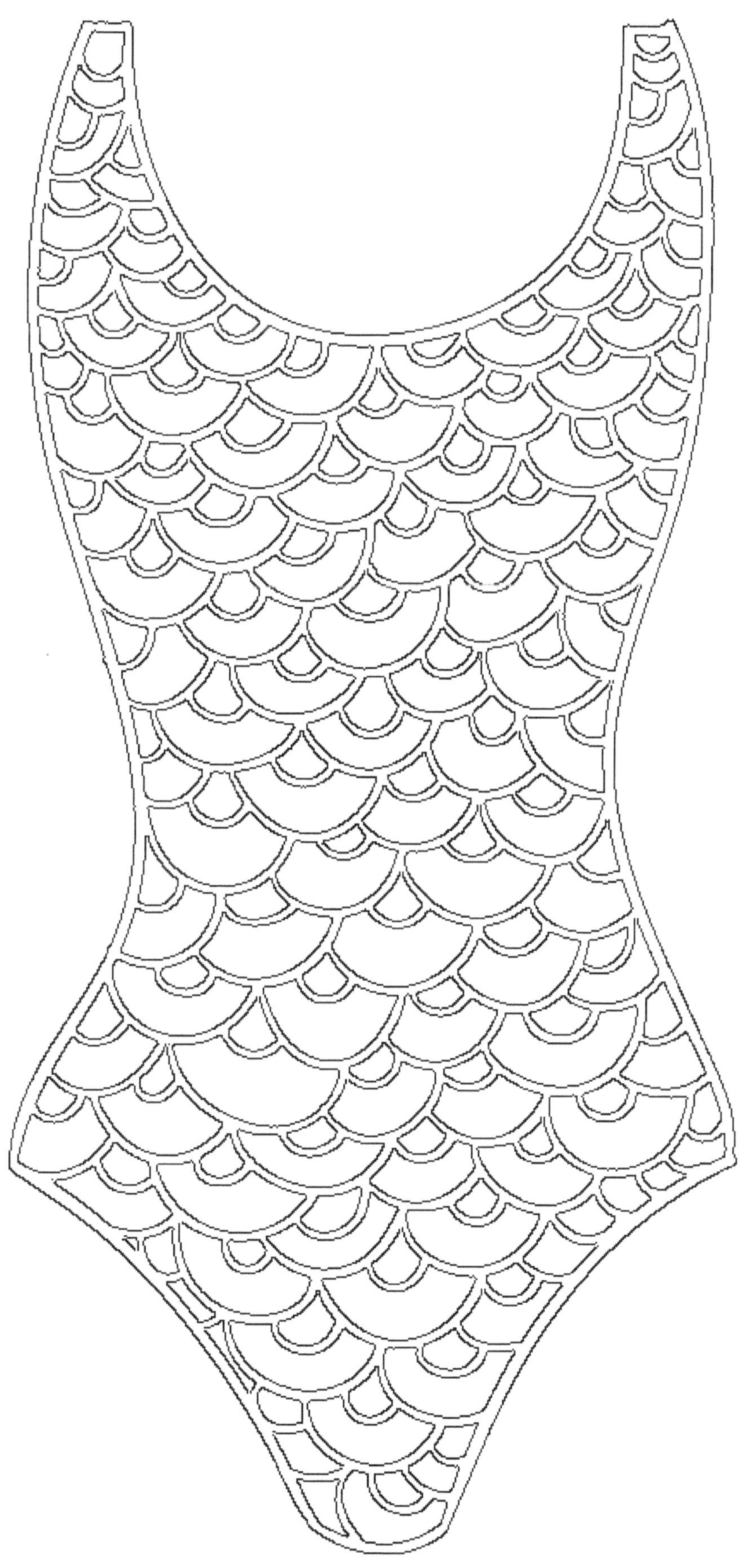

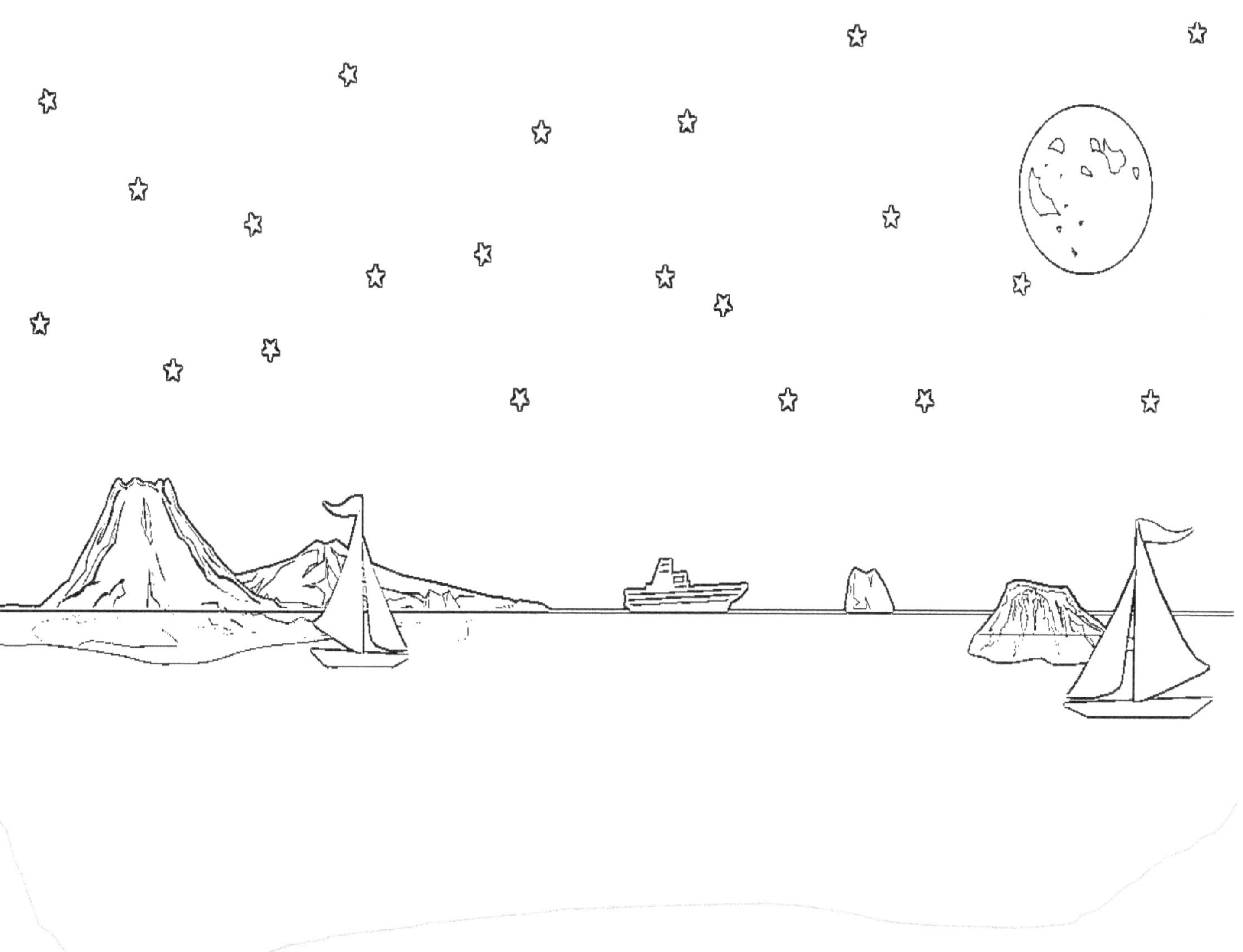

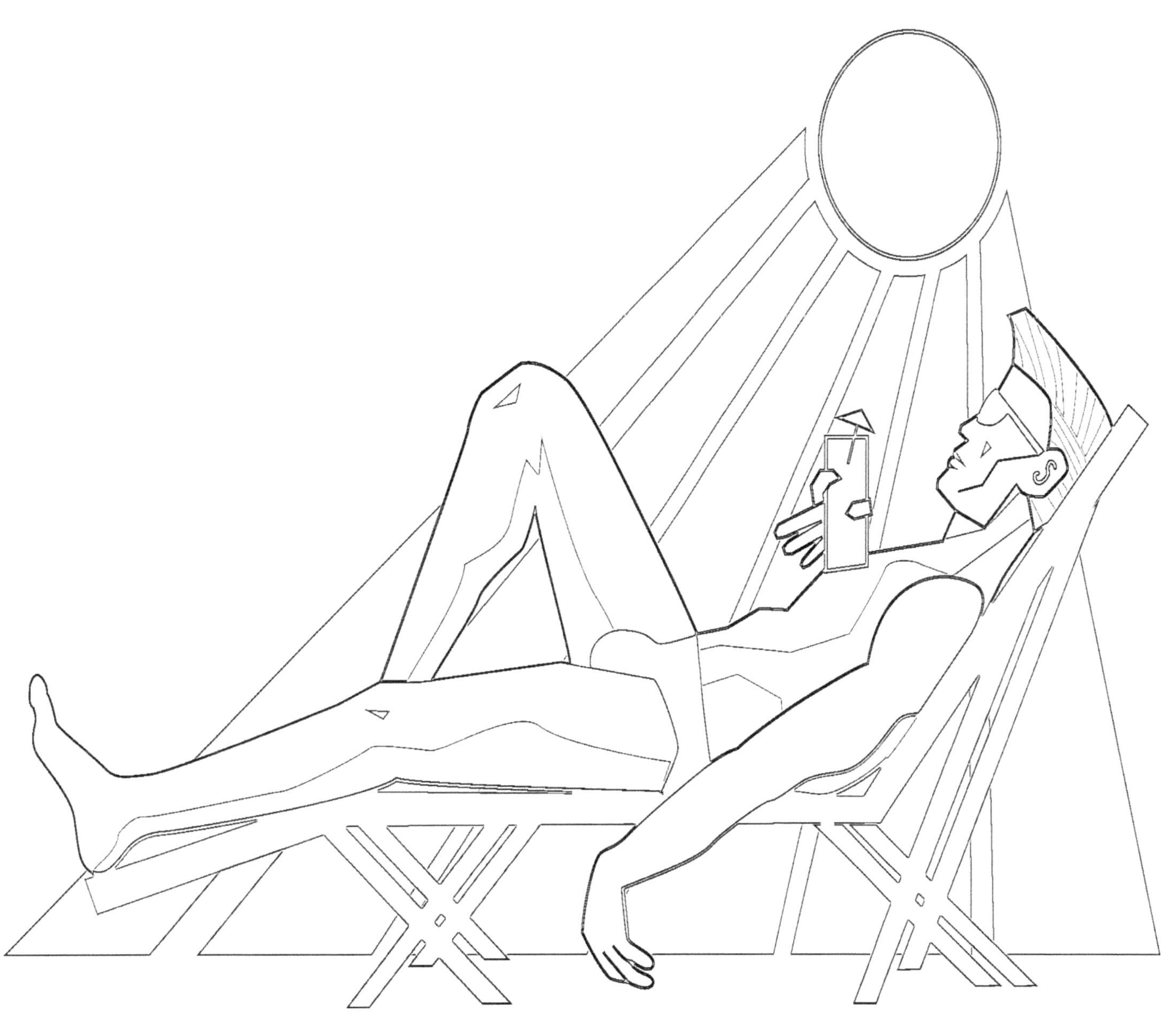

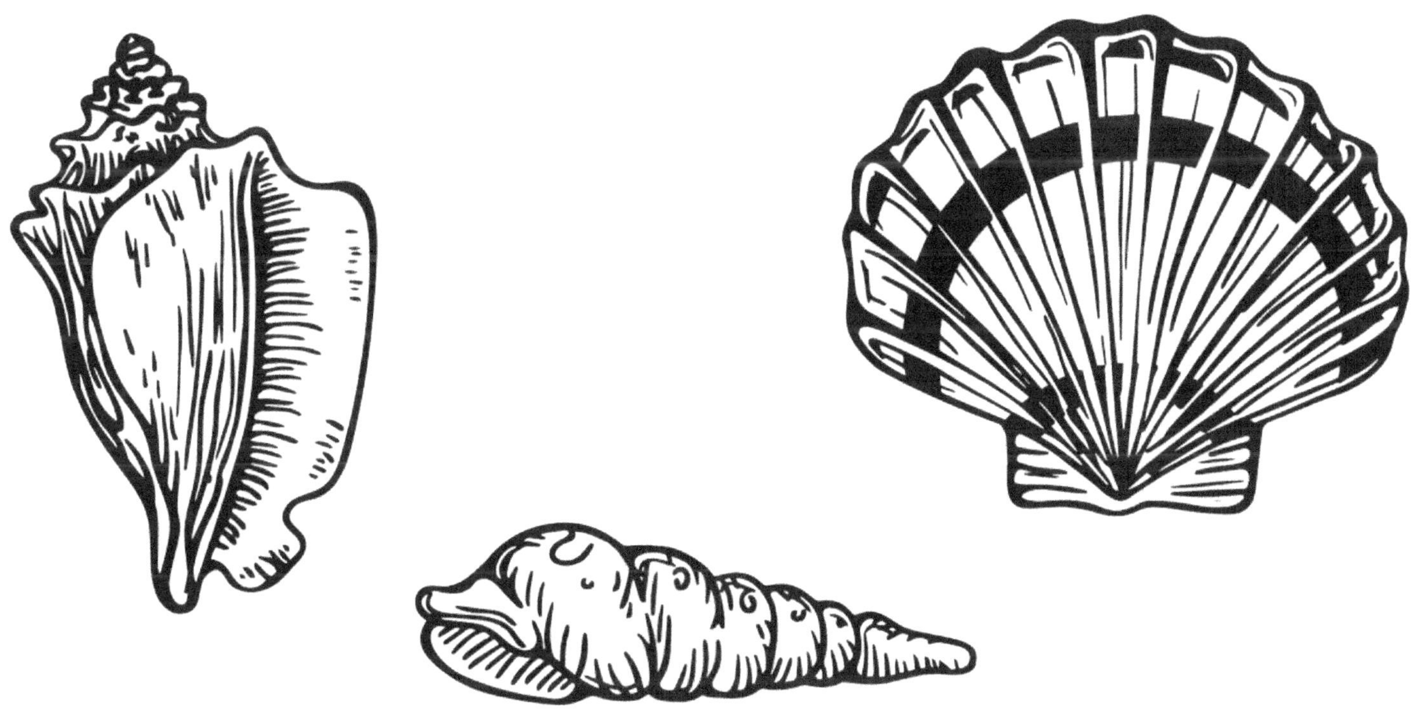

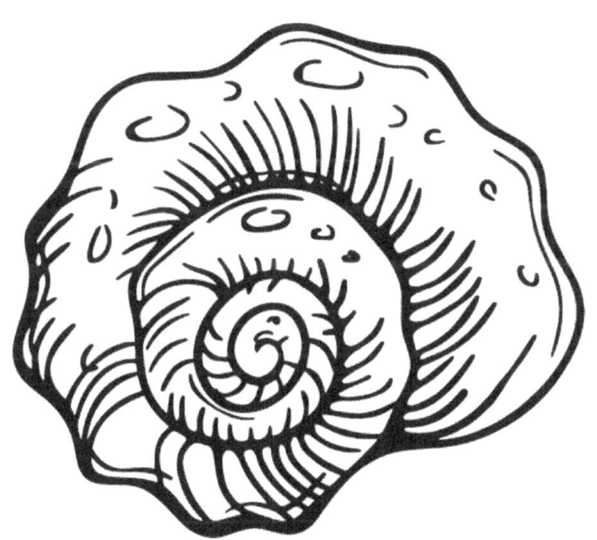

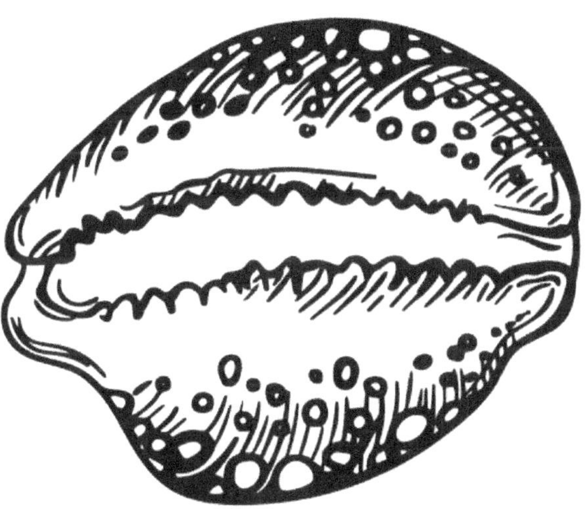

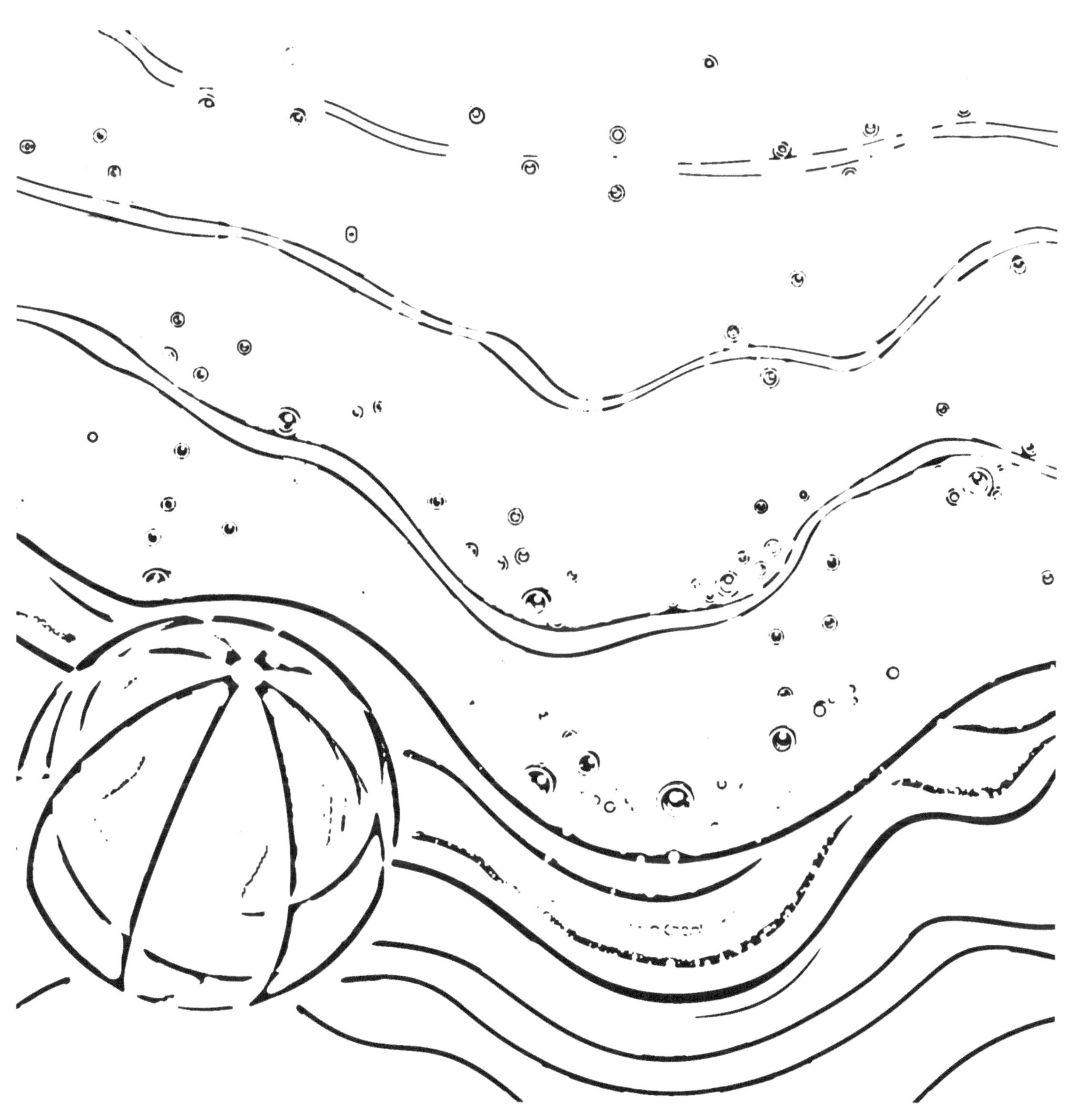

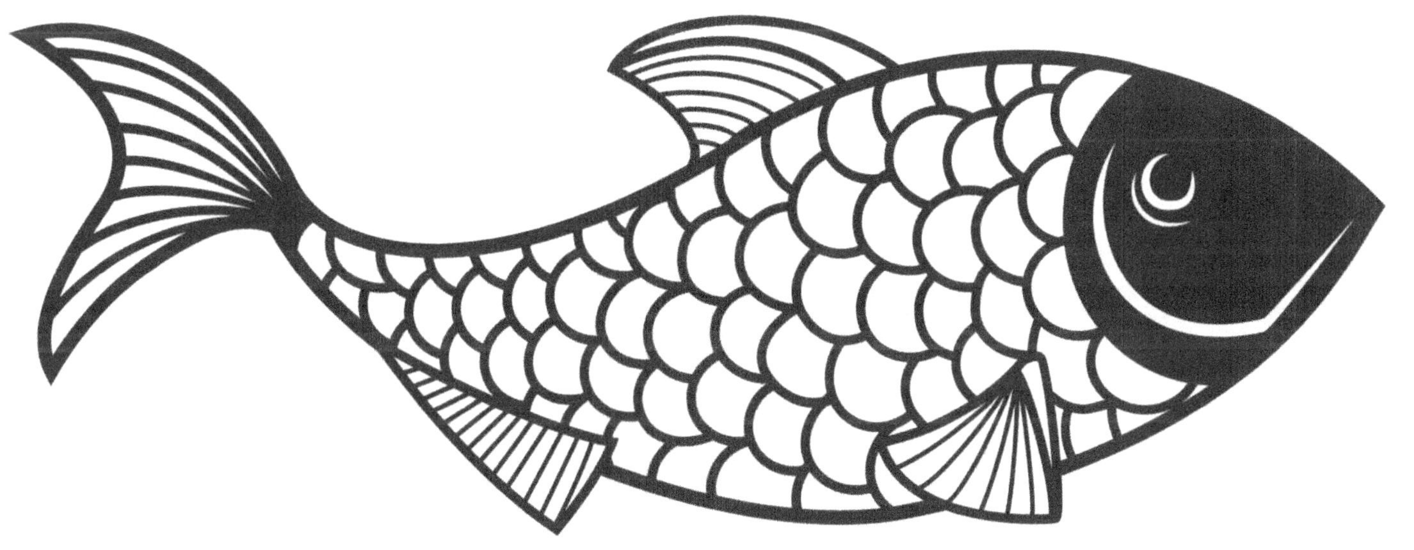

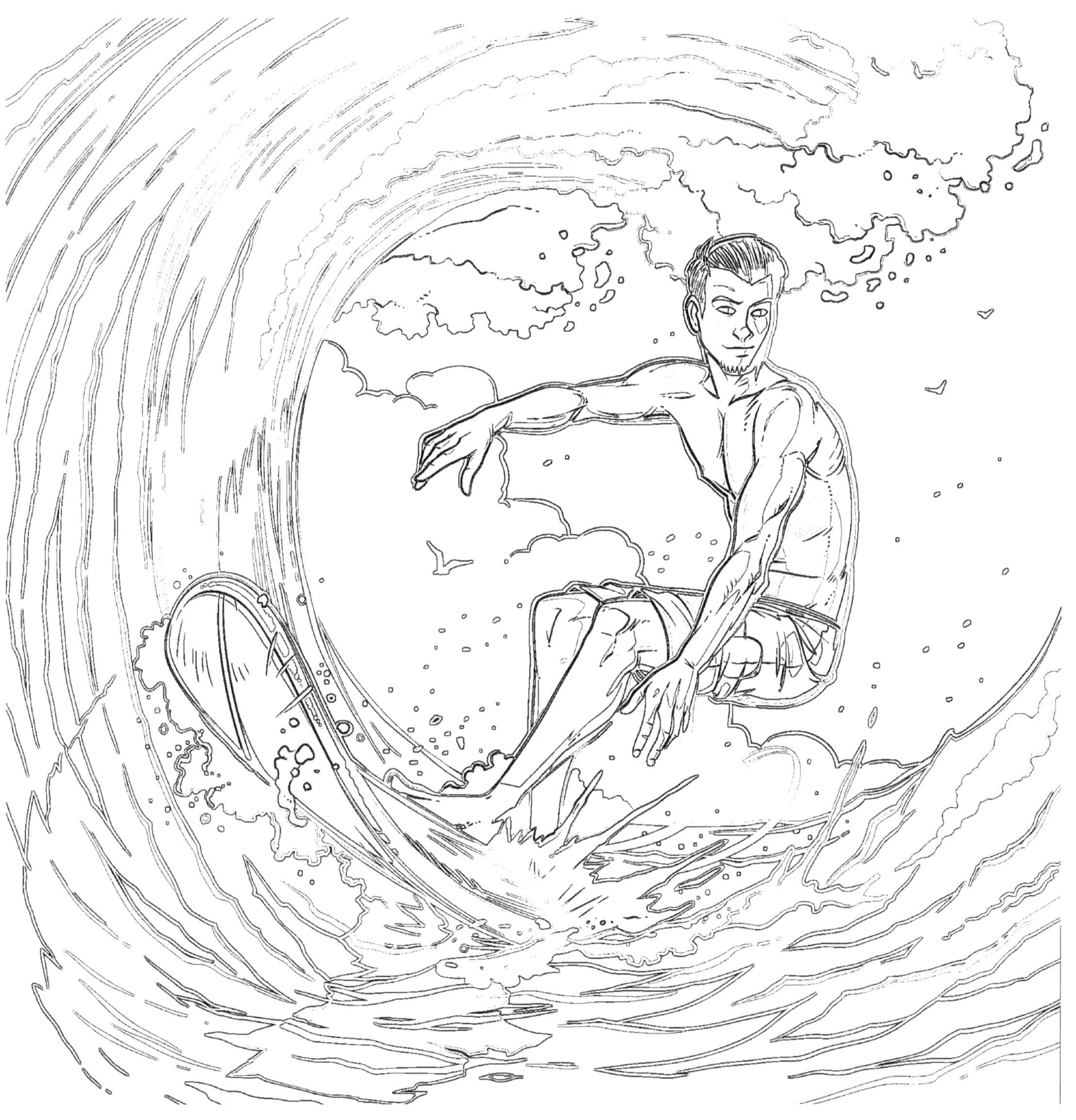

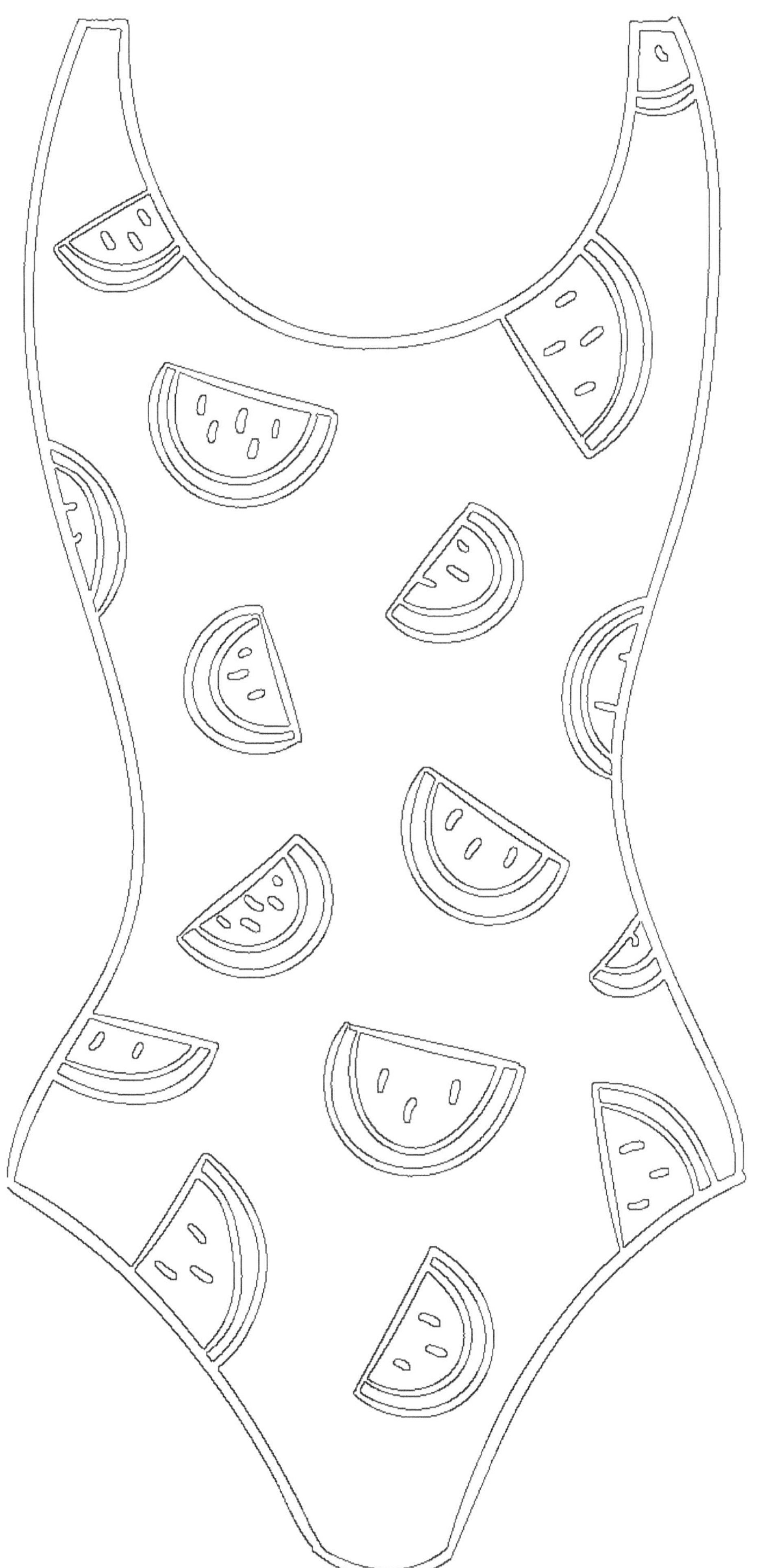

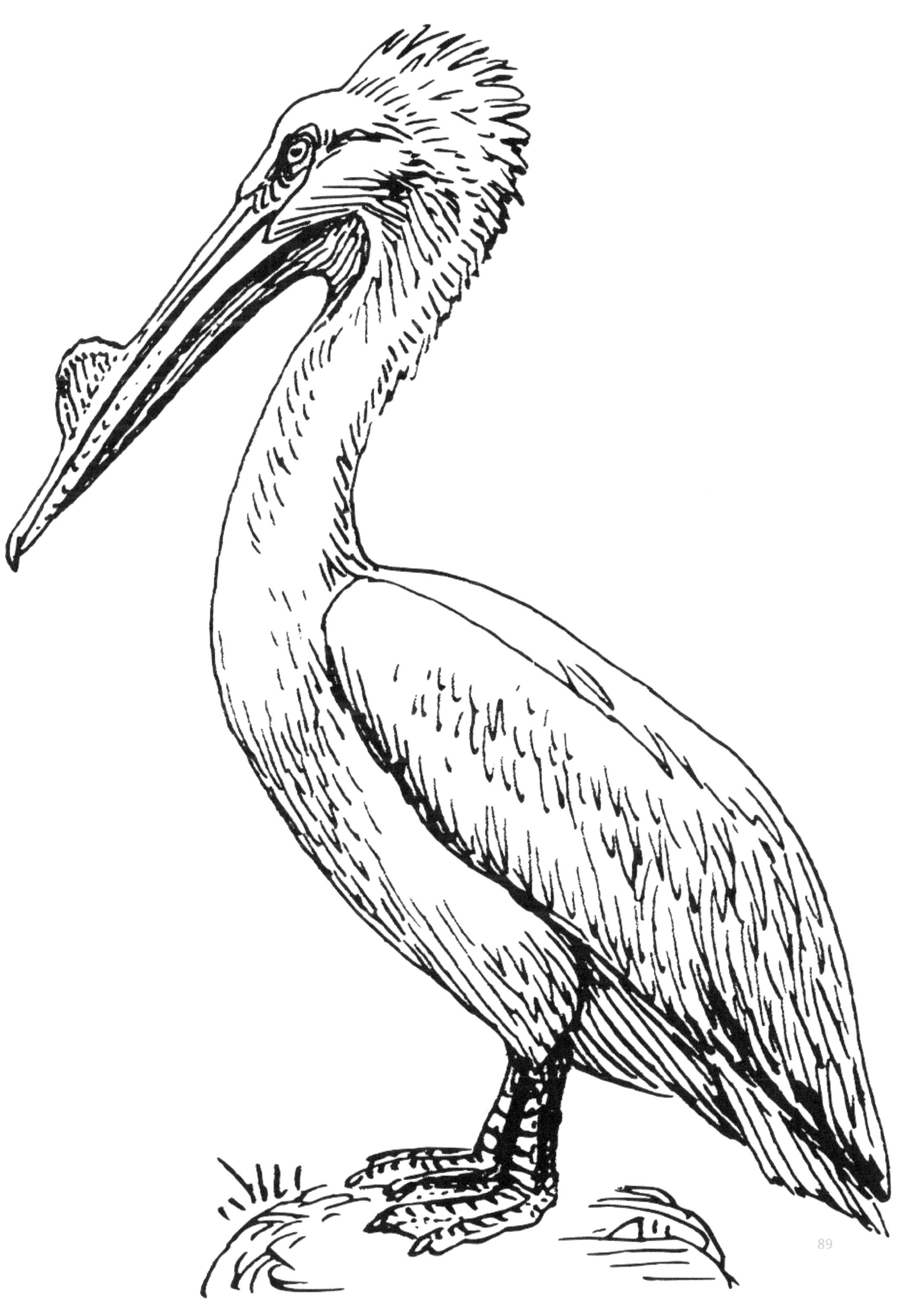

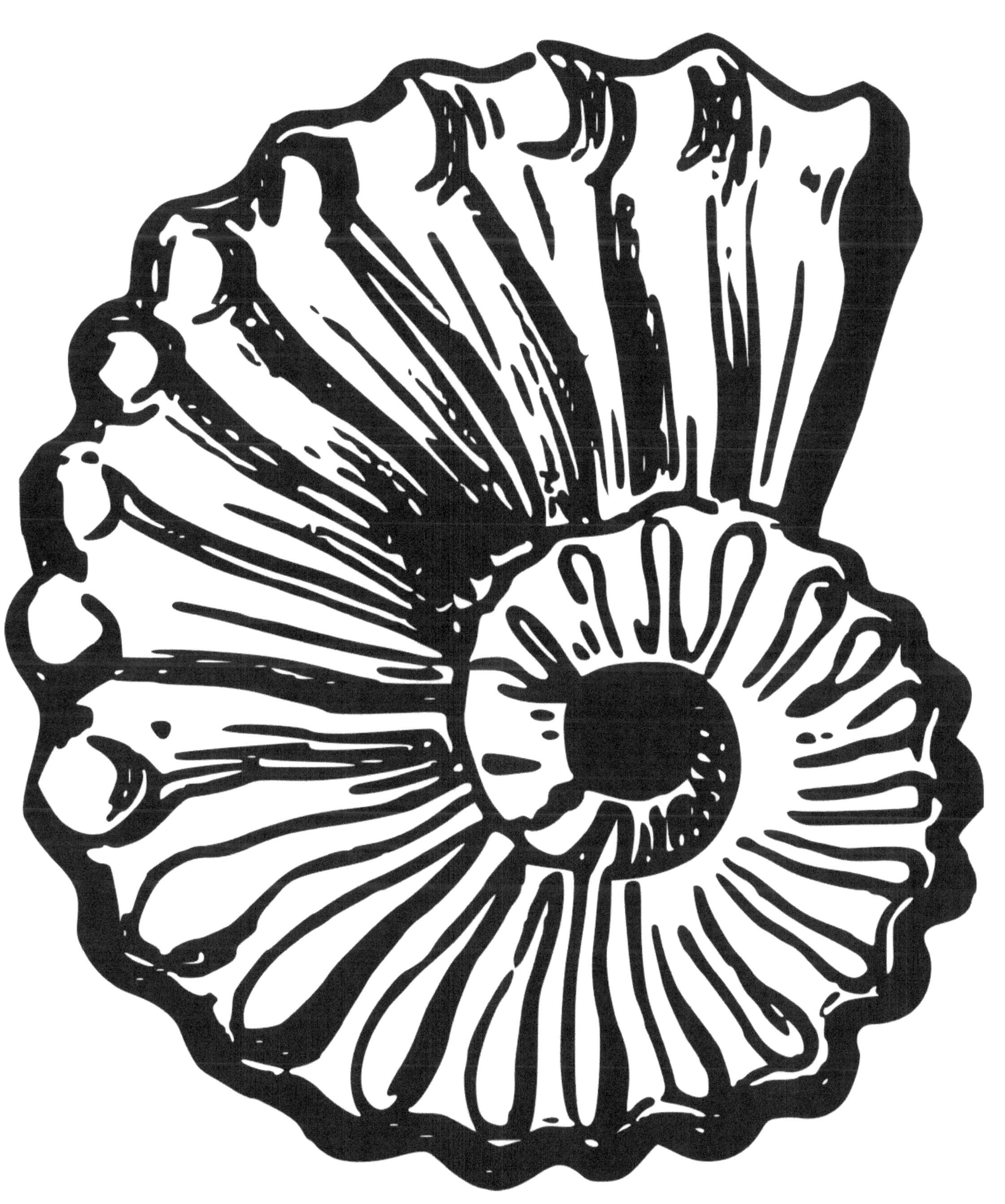

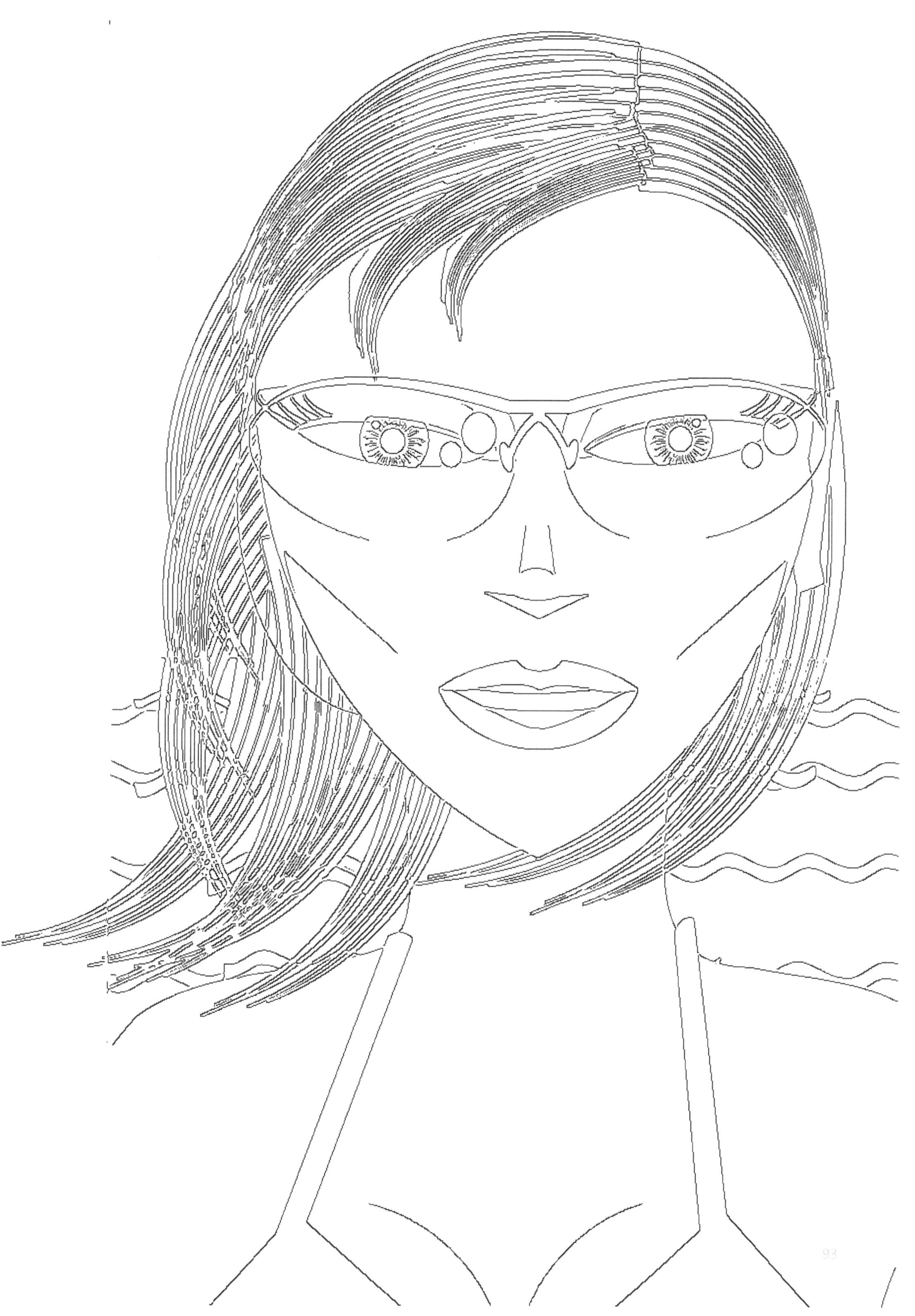

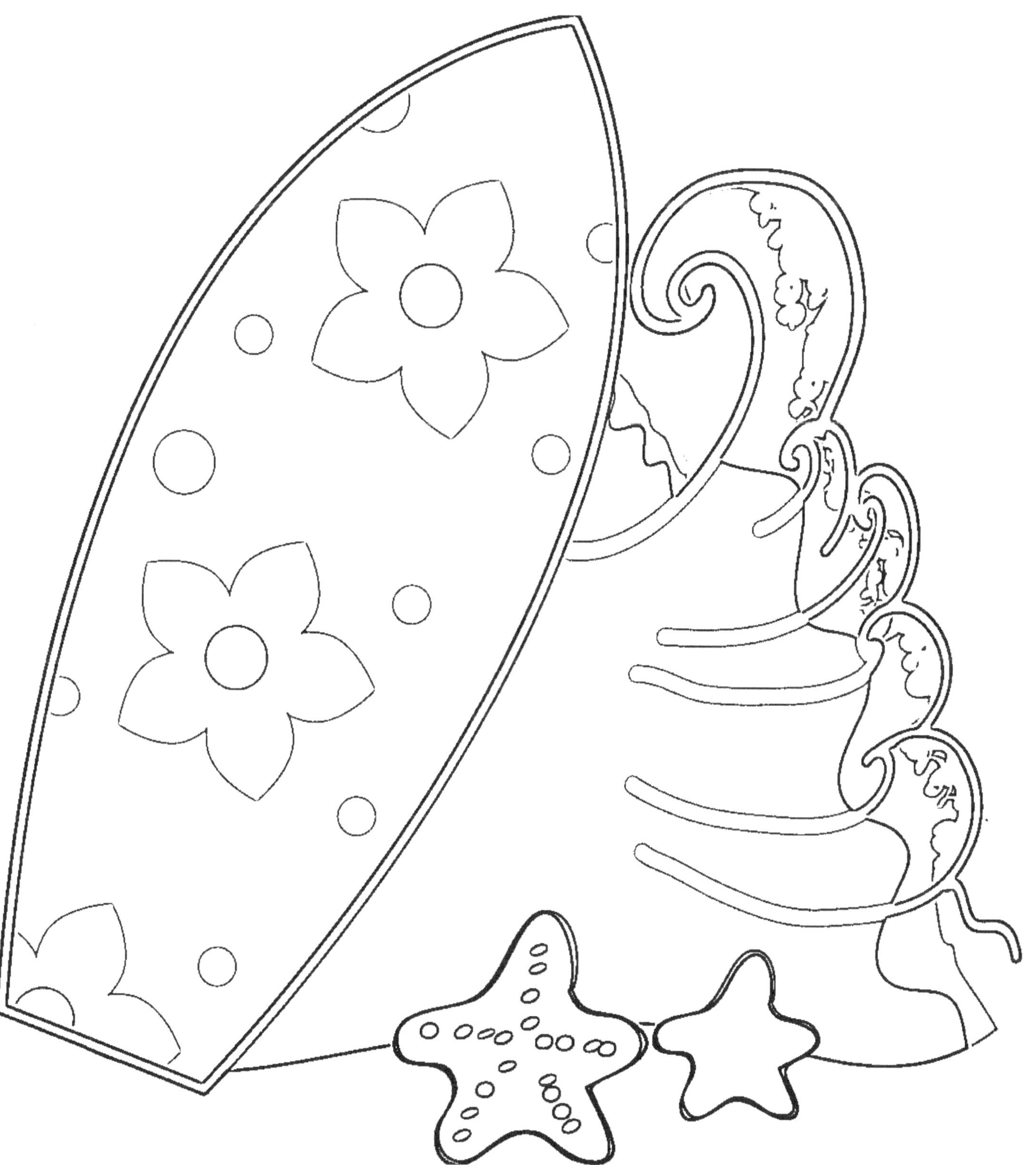

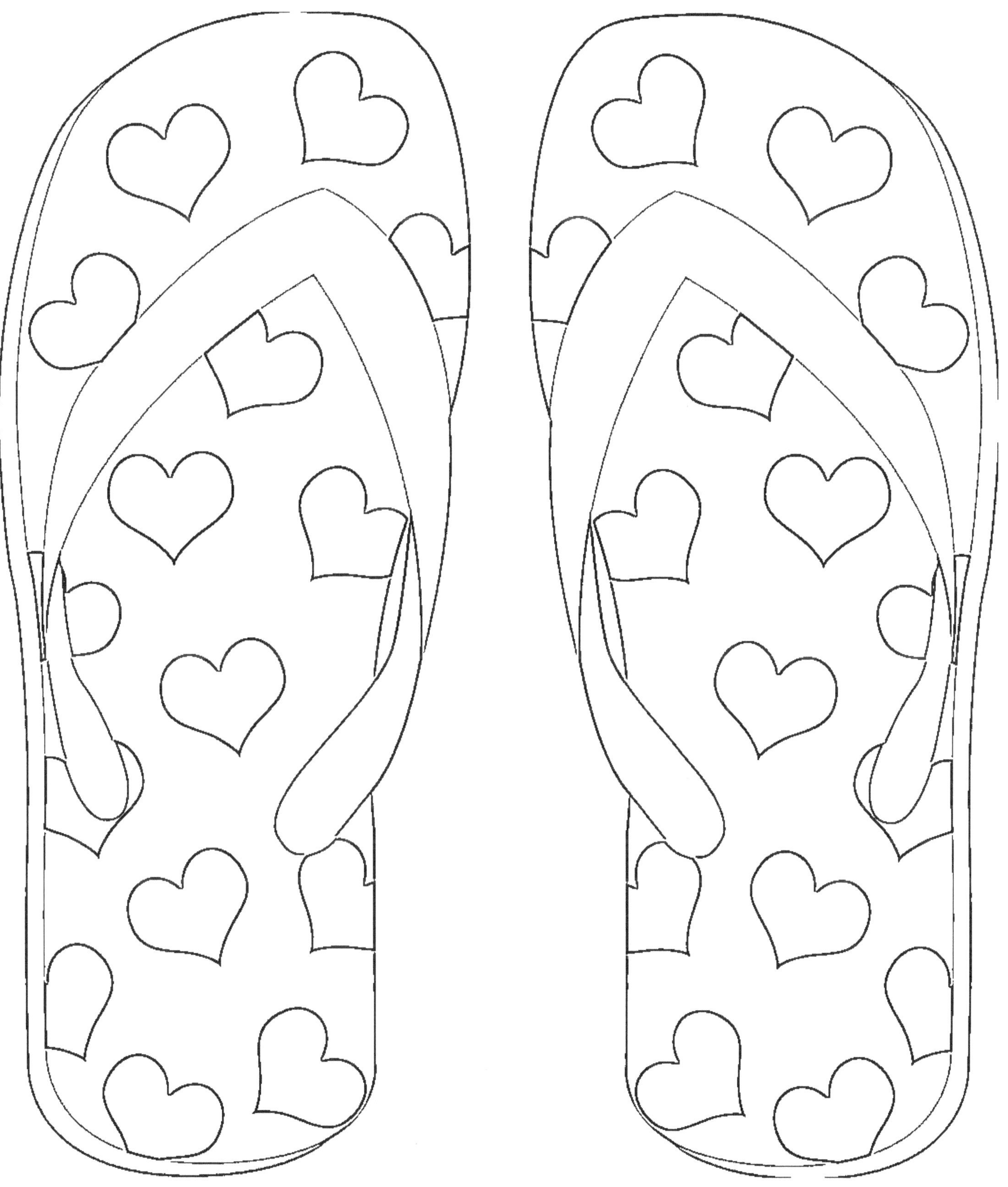

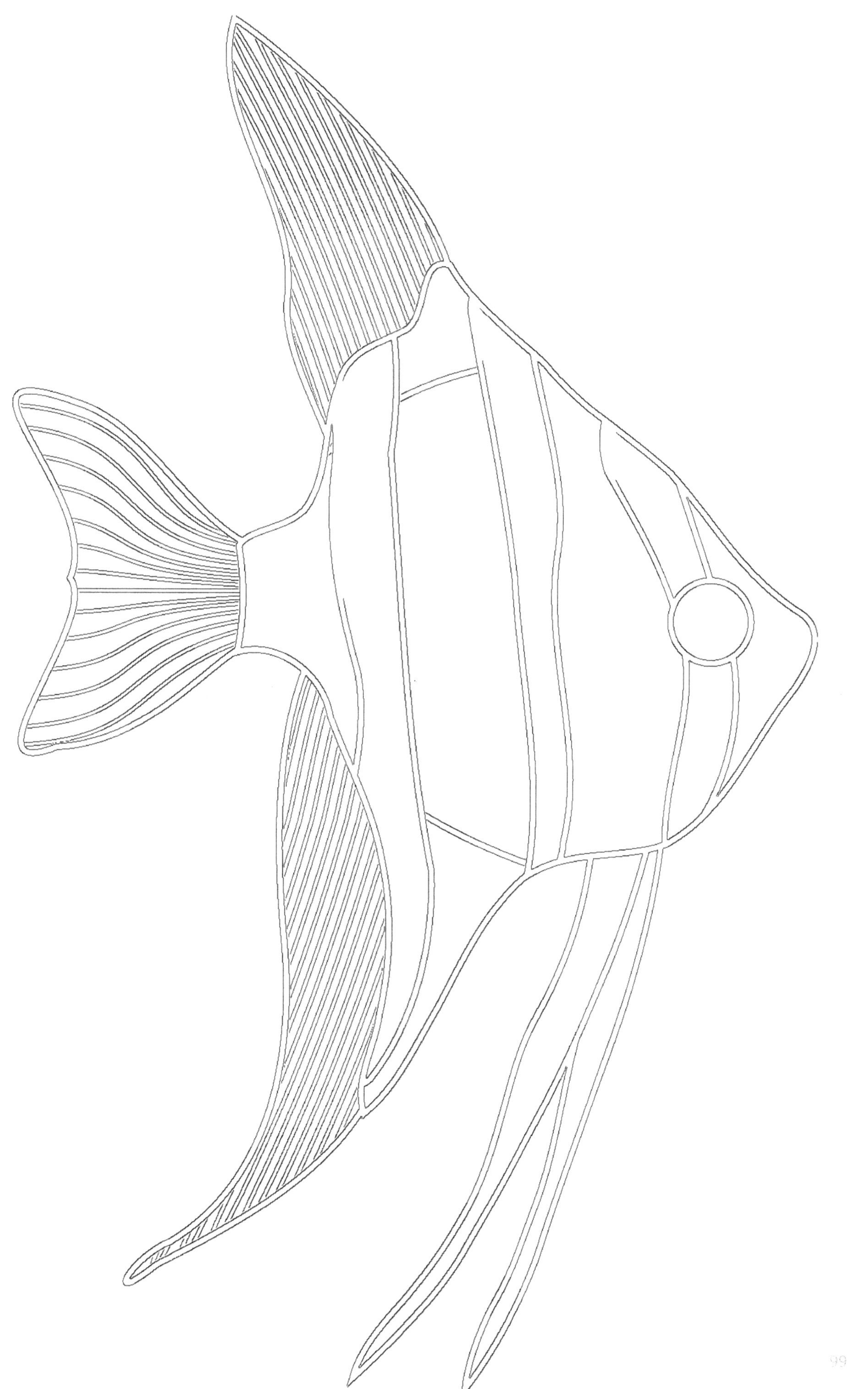

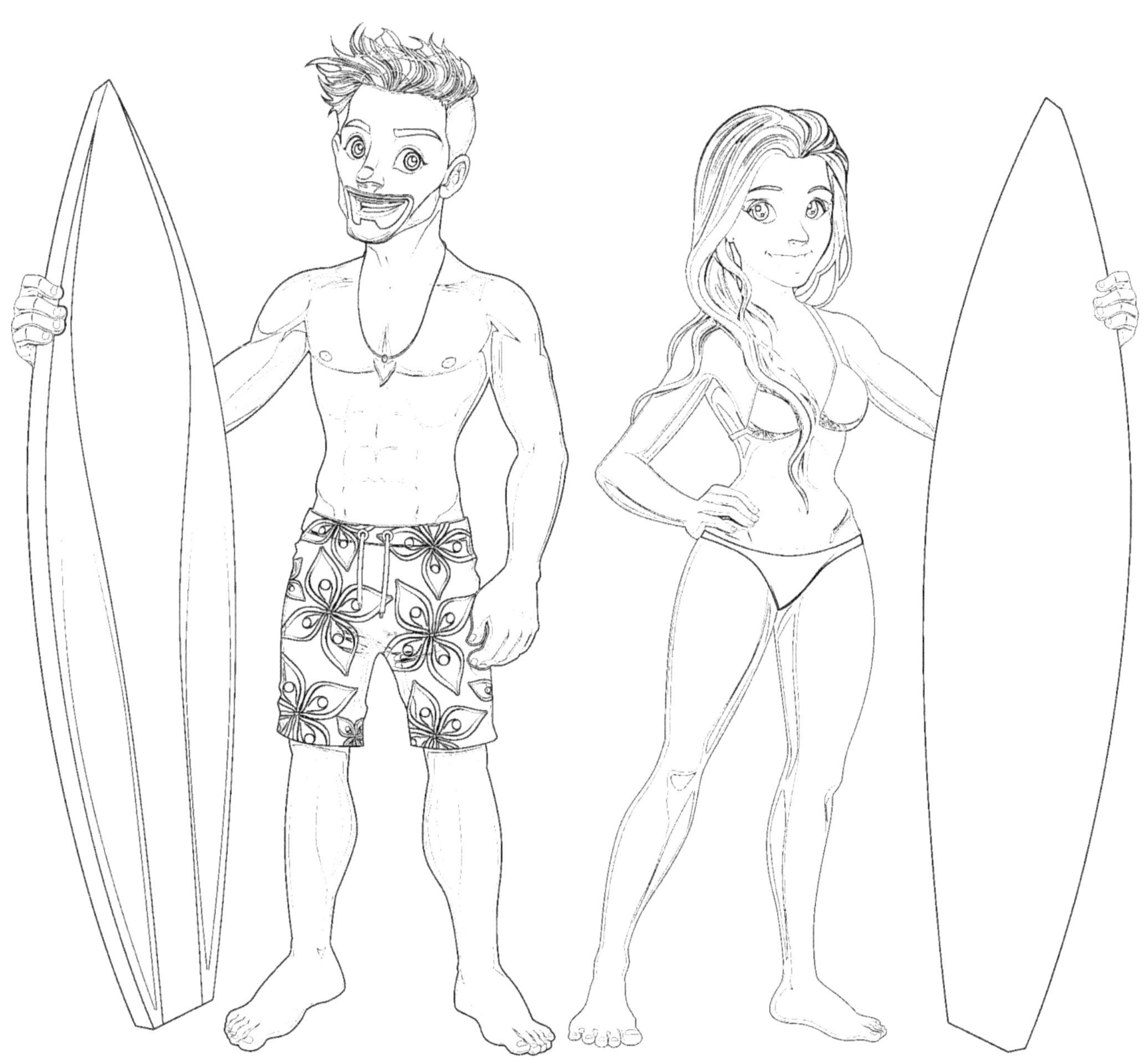

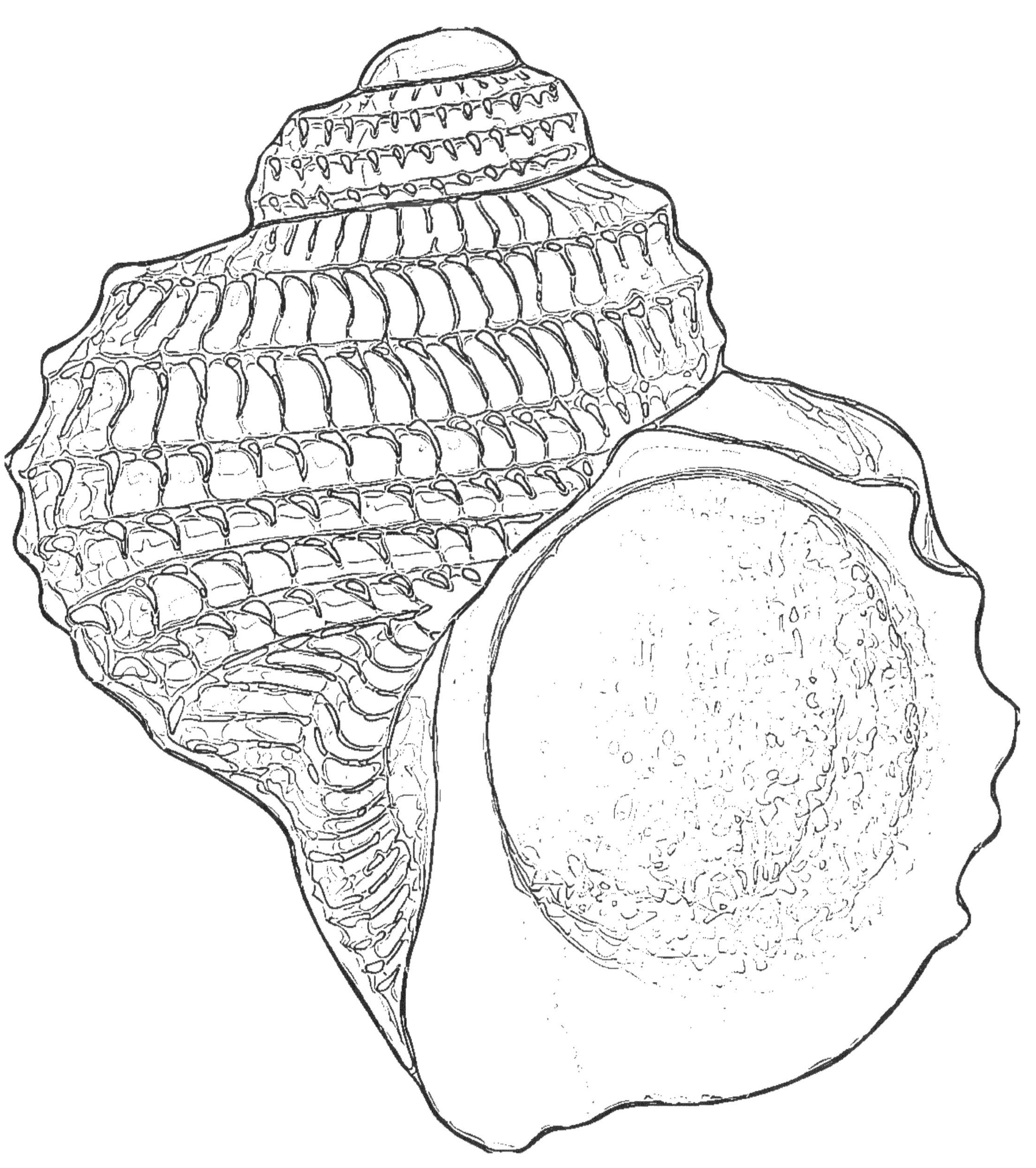

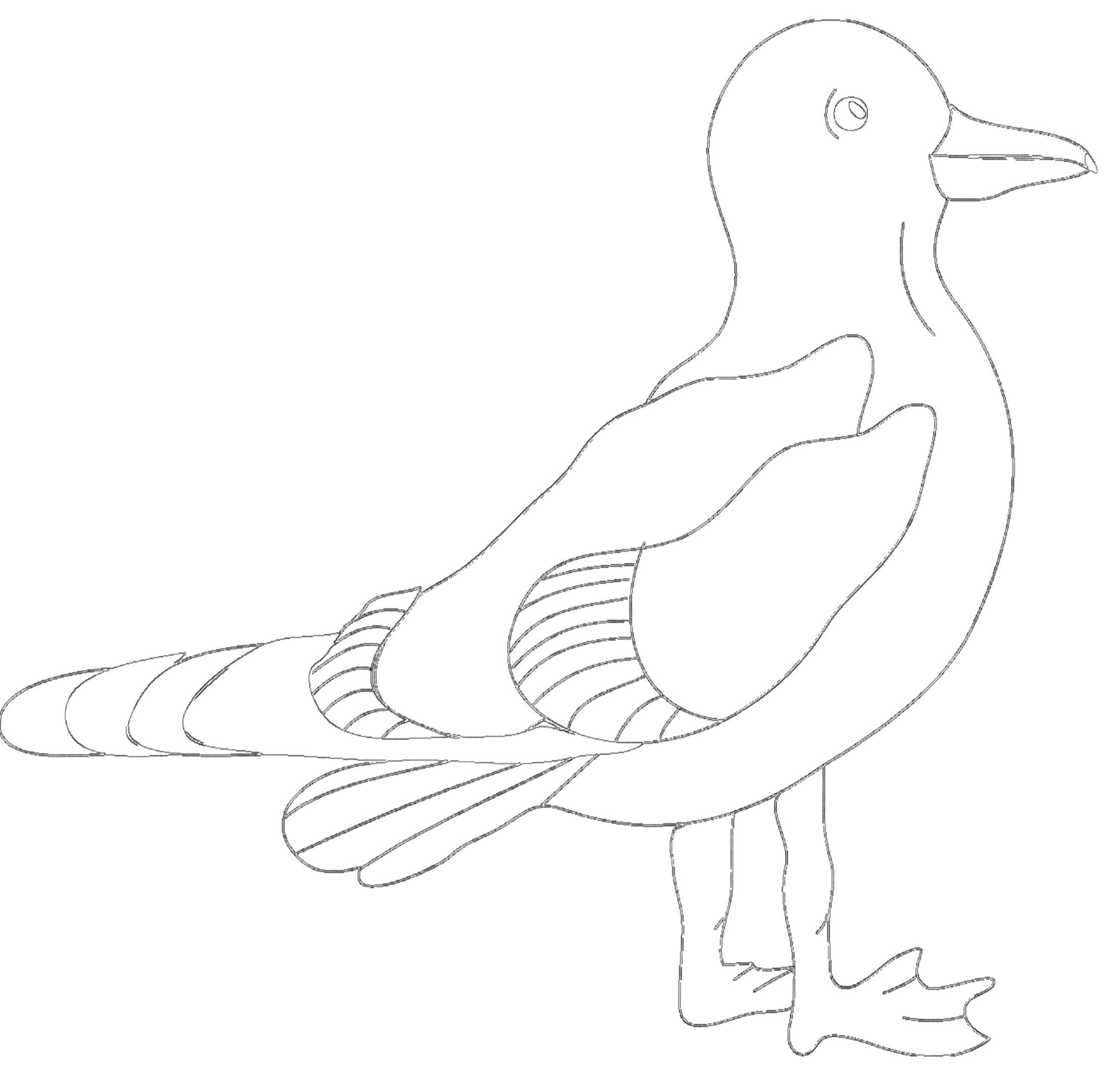

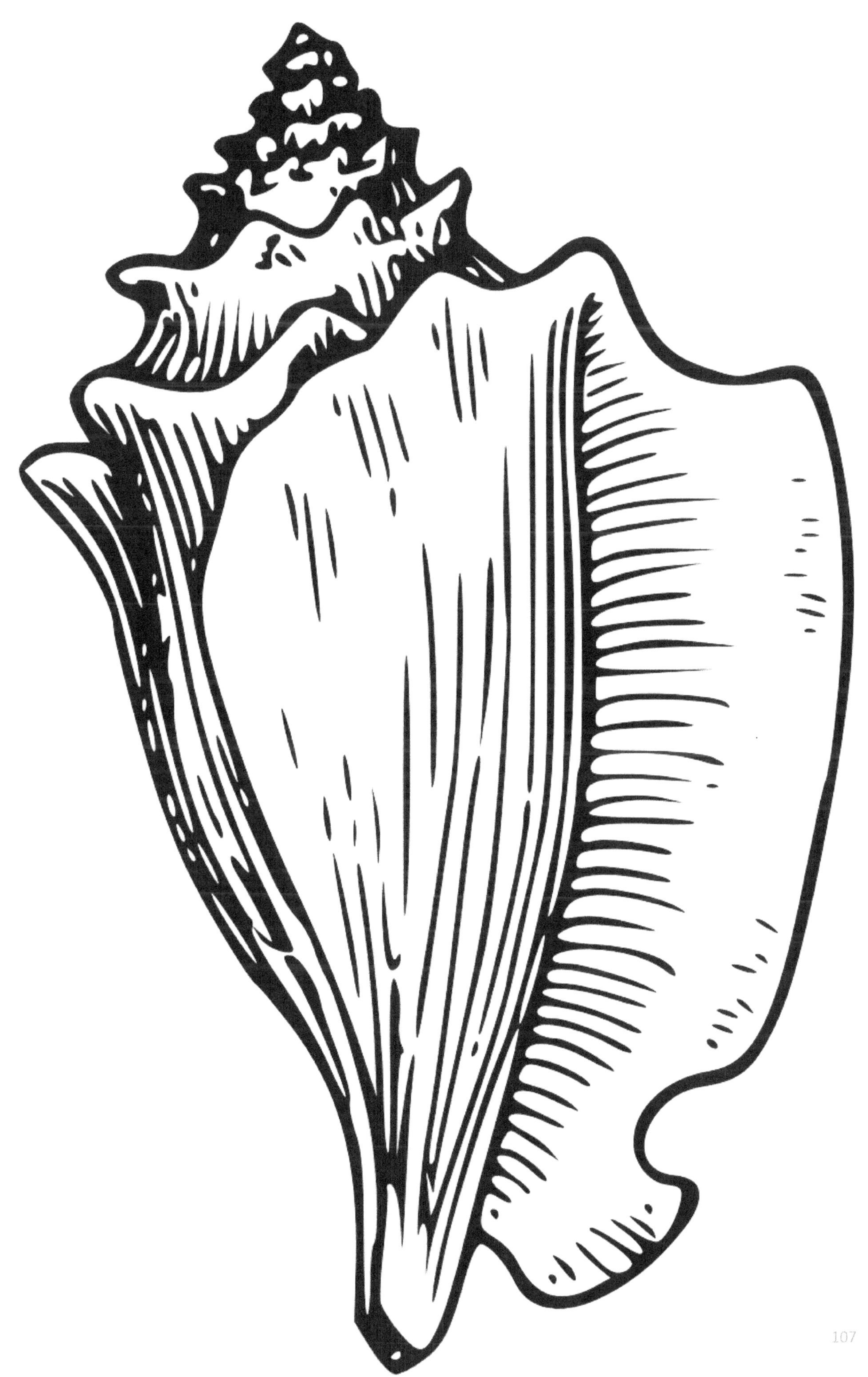

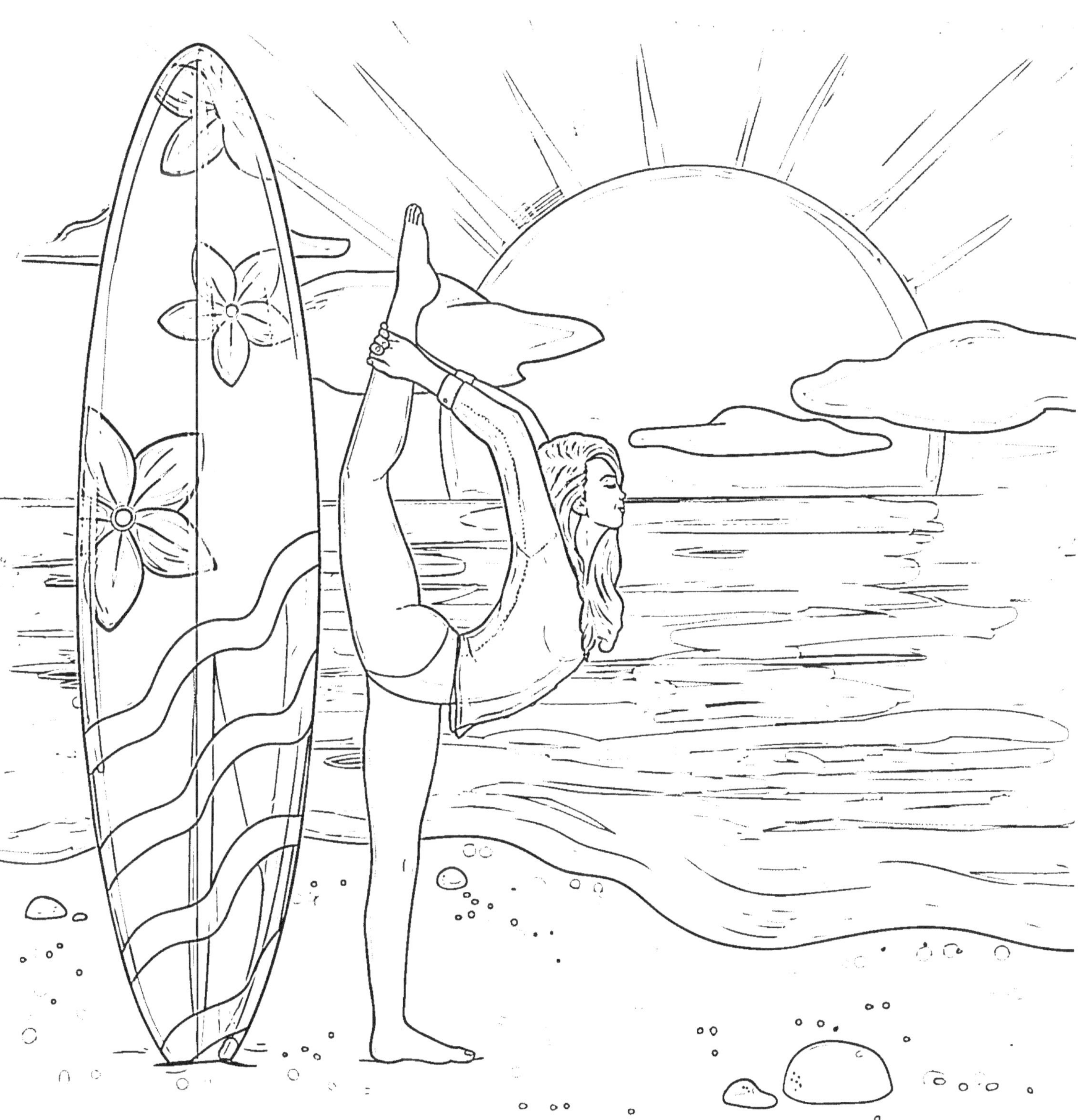